GROWING CANNABIS

A Beginner's Guide to Cultivating and Consuming Marijuana for Recreational or Medical Use

By Tom Gordon

© **Copyright 2020 - All rights reserved.**

The content contained within this book may not be reproduced, duplicated or transmitted without direct written permission from the author or the publisher.

Under no circumstances will any blame or legal responsibility be held against the publisher, or author, for any damages, reparation, or monetary loss due to the information contained within this book. Either directly or indirectly.

Legal Notice:

This book is copyright protected. This book is only for personal use. You cannot amend, distribute, sell, use, quote or paraphrase any part, or the content within this book, without the consent of the author or publisher.

Disclaimer Notice:

Please note the information contained within this document is for educational and entertainment purposes only. All effort has been executed to present accurate, up to date, and reliable, complete information. No warranties of any kind are declared or implied. Readers acknowledge that the author is not engaging in the rendering of legal, financial, medical or professional advice. The content within this book has been derived from various sources. Please consult a licensed professional before attempting any techniques outlined in this book.

GROWING CANNABIS

By reading this document, the reader agrees that under no circumstances is the author responsible for any losses, direct or indirect, which are incurred as a result of the use of information contained within this document, including, but not limited to, — errors, omissions, or inaccuracies.

GROWING CANNABIS

Table of Contents

Introduction v

Chapter One - What is Cannabis? 1

Chapter Two - Understanding the Plant 18

Chapter Three - Where to Grow Your Marijuana 34

Chapter Four - Germination of Seeds 51

Chapter Five - What Is a Mother Plant? 64

Chapter Six - Cloning Your Plants 72

Chapter Seven - Harvesting Your Crop 86

Chapter Eight - Maintenance and Preventative Control ... 106

Chapter Nine - Common Mistakes to Avoid 128

Final Words 133

INTRODUCTION

Marijuana used to be considered the product of nightmares. Everyone's favorite cartoon characters from the 1980s spoke about the dangers of marijuana. But within the last twenty years, more research than ever has been done on cannabis and the results tell a different story. While it remains true that there are ill side effects when it comes to marijuana use, the benefits have been shown to far outweigh the negatives when considered across the board, especially when considered next to caffeine, nicotine, and alcohol, all of which have been perfectly legal for years. All of the benefits of cannabis consumption have pushed North America closer and closer towards coast-to-coast legalization. In the United States, there are eleven states that allow recreational marijuana use over the age of twenty-one and thirty-three states that allow marijuana use for medical purposes. Canada legalized marijuana in October, 2018, and added more than $8 billion dollars to their GDP as a result. With legalization spreading, many people are thinking about cultivating their own plants but don't know where to start.

That's where this book comes in. In *Growing Cannabis: A Beginner's Guide to Cultivating Marijuana*, you have everything you need to know to get started growing your own cannabis. We'll first start by taking a look at the history of cannabis, its side effects, and the benefits of using it. We'll follow this up with a look at the plants themselves to understand how marijuana comes in strains and is roughly divided into two types: sativa and indica.

Following this deep dive into cannabis, we'll look at where we grow our plants. Growing marijuana indoors leads to different results than growing it outside. Which of these techniques is right for you will be left for you to decide. Once we have our setup in place, we'll turn our attention towards the seeds and see how we germinate them. This will bring us to look at what are called "mother plants" and how we use these plants in cloning. Don't worry, it's not nearly as sci-fi as it sounds.

From cloning, we'll move into harvesting to learn the best practices for harvesting the fruits of our labor. The book will then close out with a discussion on how to maintain your crops and prevent pests, fungus, or molds, as well as some tips on avoiding the common mistakes new growers seem prone to making. By the end, you will have all the knowledge you need to grow your own crop and avoid the costly pitfalls that trap less-prepared gardeners.

CHAPTER ONE

WHAT IS CANNABIS?

While marijuana certainly made its biggest impact in the last few decades, mankind has had a relationship with the cannabinoid plant family since well before recorded history. In fact, evidence dates man's discovery of the cannabis plant back to the Stone Age, around 8,000 BCE, with some scholars pointing even further back to 10,000 BCE. The history of marijuana is utterly fascinating—it takes you throughout history and all over the globe. In this chapter, we'll briefly look at the history of the cannabis plant, but our attention is primarily focused on the history of cannabinoid cultivation, which has changed drastically within our lifetimes and continues to do so as the laws become more lenient.

GROWING CANNABIS

The reason that marijuana has exploded in popularity in the past decade is due entirely to the increased research and attention on the plant. The main psychoactive component in cannabis is called tetrahydrocannabinol (THC), which has proven to be a much more interesting chemical than previously thought as much of the original research that showed us marijuana was harmful was in fact quite flawed. One of the most famous examples of this is the idea that marijuana kills brain cells. The study that came to this conclusion did so by strapping a gas mask onto a chimp and blasting it with marijuana smoke. The problem with this experiment's setup is that researchers didn't give the subject air, just smoke. Brain cells start to die when they cannot get air, regardless of what kind of smoke is being inhaled. Results like these have been proven to be scare tactics founded on faulty science, and there are actually many benefits to using marijuana responsibly. However, honest science has shown that marijuana does have some negative side effects. In order to give you a fair and accurate look at this controversial plant, we'll look at both the benefits and the risks of marijuana in this chapter.

A History of Cannabis Cultivation

While Asia has been identified as the location of origin for marijuana, it is uncertain whether the plant came out of China, Central Asia, or South Asia. In addition, many strains find their genetic roots trace back to Afghanistan and the Hindu Kush mountains (which is the reason why many strains have Kush in their names). Nevertheless, the earliest sign of cannabis cultivation comes from China between 8,000 BCE and 6,000 BCE. Evidence points to the Chinese of this period having a strong relationship with the plant, using it in many aspects of their daily lives. The hemp from the plant was used in textile production, the seeds were used as food, and even the oil seems to have been harvested for use. The Chinese are considered the inventors of farming, and one of the earliest emperors, Shennong, is credited as the inventor of many early farming tools. Shennong published one of the oldest known medical texts, and in this text, lists cannabis as a medicinal herb.

What this tells us is that from the very beginning of mankind's history with cannabis, we have been aware of its many benefits from its use in industry to its medicinal value. In an intriguing piece of contemplation, Carl Sagan considered the possibility that cannabis was the earliest crop cultivated by man. If this were so, then marijuana directly contributed to the invention of farming and our subsequent agricultural revolution. Whether Sagan's suggestion is true is yet to be seen, but the idea does present just how important cannabis cultivation has been to mankind.

Scythians, a nomadic culture from Central Asia, traded for cannabis seeds around 1,500 BCE and thereafter began to cultivate their own crops. In 600 BCE, Persia discovered cannabis. They referred to it as "bhang," or "the good narcotic." Persia's discovery of cannabis brought the plant into contact with the rest of the known world, as hemp rope can be traced to Russia in this same period. Persia's conflicts with Greek introduced the plant into post-Homeric Greece. While it is not clear exactly when or where the Roman Empire encountered cannabis, the plant made its way into their society in roughly the same period that the calendar changed over to the common era (CE). The Vikings failed to cultivate the herb in Norway and Iceland upon first discovery, but in time they managed to produce strains that could survive the cold. As a possible consequence, the Vikings may bear responsibility for bringing cannabis to North America. At the same time, the Arabs were discovering the plant. By the 14th century, cannabis was in Africa. If the Vikings hadn't brought marijuana to North America prior, then the Spanish shipped it to North America and Chile in the late 16th century. With cannabis having spread across the globe, this brings us into issues of modern cultivation.

In what is a complete mirror of the 1980s, one of the first rules related to cultivating marijuana was set by King Henry VIII, who fined farmers that would not grow the plant. Henry VII recognized the high value of

GROWING CANNABIS

hemp fibers from the plant and sought to grow as much of it as possible to fuel trade. In America, an early law required farmers to grow Indian and English hemp in their fields. Hemp cultivation in the United States was particularly fruitful thanks to ideal growing conditions. Later, the 19th century saw cannabis cultivated more for medical reasons than for its hemp. However, despite America's early relationship with the plant, laws first aimed at restricting the use of opium would grow to encompass alcohol and marijuana use with the cultivation of the latter becoming illegal. The controlled substances act of the 1970s further criminalized the substance and Nixon's War on Drugs effectively destroyed the public image of marijuana.

Despite the legalities involved, people continued to grow cannabis all over the world and even in America. However, the main source of cultivation came from strict laws designed to produce hemp or provide researchers with enough of the plant to carry out research. That research, which rediscovered marijuana's possible benefits, has led to a resurgence of cannabinoid popularity, and this popularity, backed by science, has led to changes in many of the laws around marijuana use and growth. Depending on where you live in North America today, it may still be illegal to possess or grow cannabis. Or, it may be legal to possess but not to grow cannabis. It may also be legal to grow these plants up to a certain amount, or you may even be able to get permits to grow crops for distribution to pharmacies. One thing is becoming clearer every day: Marijuana cultivation is on the rise and the laws are changing to reflect its growing popularity. Still, when it comes to growing your own marijuana, always check the laws of your country, state, and county to ensure that you stay on the side of legality.

Side Effects of Using Marijuana

Many advocates for marijuana use claim (and even believe) that there are no harmful or negative effects associated with cannabis. It would be amazing if such a claim was true, but the reality and science indicates that there are negative effects associated with marijuana use and users should be aware of them. However, it is worth noting that some of these negative effects may, depending on the user's circumstances, in fact, be positive. For example, some people may see increased appetite as a negative side effect, but for someone having trouble with nausea or eating (due to, say, the effects of chemotherapy), this side effect would be a positive.

GROWING CANNABIS

When smoking or consuming marijuana, there are a number of associated short-term effects collectively referred to as the "high." These effects include distorted perception, and the user's sights, sounds, time, or touch may seem slightly off. Issues with coordination, memory, and learning all present as side effects as well. Likewise, the user may find reductions in their critical thinking and problem solving abilities. An increased heart rate is also common. These effects in and of themselves are quite often the user's goals. For example, the distorted perception can make viewing movies or listening to music a deeply engrossing or even spiritual experience. However, as enjoyable as these situations may be, they are still effects that the user should be aware of.

In some cases, anxiety, fear, paranoia, or even panic may be found among the short-term effects experienced by the user. The mental healths of the user and the emotions that they are feeling when they partake in marijuana have a strong influence on how the user perceives the experience. This can lead to a "bad trip" or even "greening out," in which the user experiences an upset stomach or even vomit. More often than not, this reaction is due to the psychological experience the user is having and not the physical experience of their body.

The active chemical in cannabis, THC, attaches to cannabinoid receptors found on nerve cells in the brain. The THC then has an influence on how these cells function. Different parts of the brain have different amounts of these cannabinoid receptors. Some have many, while some have none.

Unsurprisingly, the areas of the brain in which cannabinoid receptors are concentrated are those that deal with the experience of pleasure, memory, thought, concentration, perception, or movement. High doses of marijuana can cause these areas to function poorly, and in the worst experiences, this can mean hallucinations, delusions, or disorientation.

Meanwhile, while THC is attaching itself to the user's cannabinoid receptors, the effect of introducing a new chemical into the body leads to an increased heart rate. When the heart starts to beat quicker, there is a corresponding drop in blood pressure. Use of marijuana can see your heart rate increase between 20%-100%. This change in the functioning of the heart leaves users at a heightened risk of heart attack during the first hour of smoking. This increased risk is not high enough to be a major concern to the average user, but anybody that is combining medications or dealing with heart-related medical issues should be wary about consuming marijuana and consult with a physician beforehand.

Another issue which was brought into light in 2017 is marijuana's relationship with the body's bones. Studies have found that users who smoke large quantities of marijuana on a regular basis have a reduced bone density compared to light or nonsmokers. As a result, heavy marijuana smokers have greater susceptibility to fractures or broken bones. The study which discovered this also found that those users have a lower body mass index, which may be the reason for the lower bone density. However, a similar study from 2017 did not find any connection between bone density and marijuana use, which means that this finding is still up in the air and requires more research.

Smoking marijuana causes the lungs and throat to burn and can cause fits of heavy coughing. Users have for years claimed that there is no harmful effect to smoking marijuana, but a study in 2019 found that regular intake of marijuana smoke can cause similar respiratory issues to that of tobacco. A persistent cough, frequent chest illnesses, and an increased risk of lung infections are all possible side effects. Many marijuana smokers intake less smoke (volumetrically) than the average tobacco user and this can be one reason we see fewer lung issues in marijuana smokers. It is not the chemical, THC, that causes this issue, but the act of taking smoke into the lungs. One clear issue in relation to marijuana smokers is the method through which many users inhale deeply and hold the smoke in their lungs. This practice is seen as a way to increase the amount of THC entering the body, but doing so also exposes the lungs to the carcinogenic properties of the smoke for a greater period of time. However, despite the similarities between smoking marijuana and tobacco, there has not yet been any confirmed research similarly linking marijuana use to increased risk of cancer.

One other area that we need to address is the use of marijuana during pregnancy. It is never a good idea to take substances when pregnant and marijuana is no exception. Studies have found that prenatal exposure to marijuana can result in children born with strange responses to visual stimuli, increased tremulousness, issues with attention and memory, and poor problem solving skills. If you wouldn't drink while pregnant, then you shouldn't smoke while pregnant either.

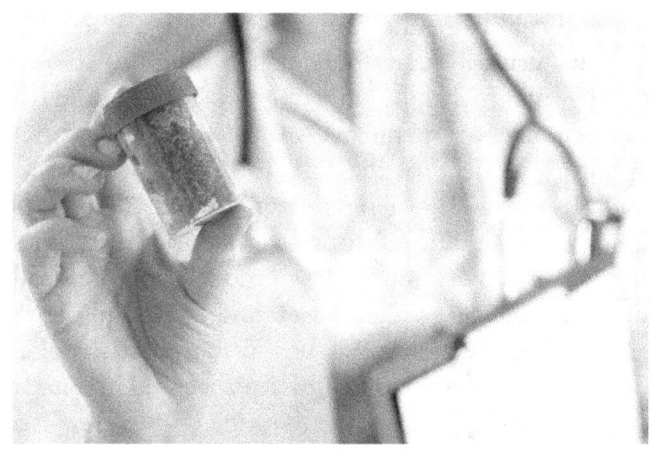

The Benefits of Marijuana Use

If everything was negative, there would be no push for the widespread legalization of marijuana. But as you will see, the benefits are many. One of the things that we should take note of here is CBD. CBD stands for cannabidiol and it is the second most common compound to marijuana after THC. While THC is the chemical which provides the "high," which can bring both positives and negatives, CBD provides no high. It does, however, offer many benefits with no evidence of harmful side effects (as of this writing). The presence of these two chemicals is important to note because growers may aim to produce marijuana with a low THC and high CBD, or a high THC and low CBD, or any combination thereof. What this means for us is that the benefits associated with marijuana may be different depending on the particular strain discussed. We'll look at the importance of strains in the next chapter, but for our purposes here, we'll look at the overall agreed-upon benefits that marijuana can have.

The cannabinoids in marijuana have been shown to be of benefit in managing and providing relief for chronic pain. This is one of the primary reasons why cannabis has become a popular medical choice. With CBD oil, patients can find relief for their pain without having to turn to an opiate. Similarly, cannabis has been linked to a reduction in tremors and pain when taken by people with Parkinson's disease. It has also been linked to reducing the side effects of hepatitis C and the impact of negative side effects from hepatitis C treatment. There has also been compelling evidence that marijuana can offer pain relief to those with multiple sclerosis and arthritis. Cannabidiol (CBD) in particular has been linked to shortening the time the body needs to mend broken bones and reducing the pressure applied to the eyeball from glaucoma.

But that's not even close to all the benefits. Cannabis has an impact on the body's production of insulin and it has been shown to help stabilize blood sugar levels and improve blood circulation. Likewise, we saw that cannabis intake can lead to temporarily lowered blood pressure. For those suffering from high blood pressure, this effect can actually be seen as a benefit. Cannabis use has also been linked to a reduction in weight. This finding is linked to the findings on diabetes since the change in the body's insulin helps the body to more efficiently use the calories that are consumed.

There is a ton of research showing that cannabis can help to fight certain kinds of cancer. This is the most controversial of the benefits and should not be blown out of proportion. Marijuana use has been linked to an improvement and reduction in cancer in patients but it is not in itself a cure for cancer. Taking smoke into the lungs can still cause lung cancer, even if the smoke comes from marijuana and not some other substance. However, along with these intriguing findings, there are many first-hand reports about the helpfulness of marijuana consumption in limiting nausea from chemotherapy.

Cannabis has been used to help battle alcohol addiction, though much work is still needed in this area. It has also been used to help people with Crohn's disease or ulcerative colitis to reduce inflammation in the intestines. There has been a lot of research showing that cannabis can help in the treatment of PTSD when used in conjunction with a mental health specialist. Likewise, cannabis has been shown to reduce anxiety in many users. However, people that use marijuana to treat anxiety have also reported the effects turning against them and making them more anxious, so this particular area can be either beneficial or harmful. This finding is also repeated in those looking at depression. Cannabis has also been shown to help people with ADHD focus better and has been considered as an alternative to traditional drugs such as Ritalin or Adderall.

Whether it is your mind or your body, there are many ways that the use of marijuana can be beneficial to the user. The most intriguing part of these benefits is

GROWING CANNABIS

that marijuana offers a far safer alternative to some of the scarier chemicals used medically today such as Adderall and opiates. Still, despite the many potential benefits, it is always best to consult with a medical professional before using marijuana, and it is always a good idea to start slow and see how your body reacts to cannabis.

GROWING CANNABIS

Chapter Summary

- Humanity's relationship with cannabis goes back as far as 10,000 BCE.

- The earliest signs of cannabis cultivation date to between 8,000 BCE and 6,000 BCE and come from China.

- Evidence suggests that the Chinese used cannabis on a daily basis as both a food and a medicine.

- The Chinese are also the inventors of farming, which has led some to suggest that cannabis was humanity's earliest cultivated crop.

- Cannabis spread out from Asia, making its way all over the world from Europe to Iceland, North America, and Africa.

- One of the first laws relating to cannabis was a demand by King Henry VIII to grow more. One of America's earliest laws relating to cannabis also required farmers to cultivate the plant.

- Cannabis only gained its illicit status in the 1900s due to anti-substance campaigns in the 1920s. Recent years has found its cultivation and use resurge as new research has led to changing attitudes about marijuana.

- Short-term side effects of smoking marijuana include distorted perception, issues with memory and learning, issues thinking or solving problems, and increased heart rate.

- Some people may experience fear, paranoia, panic, or anxiety after smoking cannabis.

- THC, the active chemical in cannabis, attaches to receptors in the brain to cause the effects associated with the "high" of marijuana.

- As THC attaches to the brain, the user's heart rate increases between 20%-100% leading to reduced blood pressure. If you have any heart issues, consult with a doctor before using marijuana.

- Smoking cannabis also exposes the user to the possibility of developing issues with the lungs. However, there has yet to be any confirmed link between use of cannabis and lung cancer.

- Cannabis should also not be used by pregnant women, as there are links between cannabis use and learning disabilities.

- Another active ingredient in cannabis is CBD, which helps to reduce pain and provide many benefits to users.

- High CBD strains are recommended for use in pain management as an alternative to opioids.

- Cannabis has also been linked to helping reduce tremors and pain in people suffering from Parkinson's, reduce the side effects of hepatitis

C treatment, and shorten the time it takes bones to heal.

- Cannabis has also been shown to have a positive impact on how the body uses insulin, as well as help in weight reduction for these reasons.

- There is strong evidence that cannabis use can help in preventing or battling cancer, though these findings are often treated like a magic cure. While cannabis helps in managing cancer, it does not and should not replace proper medical treatment.

- Marijuana has been used to help battle alcohol addiction, reduce anxiety and depression, and help people with ADHD to focus better.

- Every day, there are more findings about the beneficial effects of cannabis. However, there are also more findings about possible downsides to cannabis use. If you have any medication conditions, do your research and speak with your doctor about cannabis use prior to beginning.

In the next chapter, you will learn why genetics are important in growing and cultivating cannabis. You will also learn what we mean when we speak about different strains of marijuana. Finally, we'll look in depth at sativa, indica, hybrids, and ruderalis, the main varieties that the cannabis plant comes in. Each has its own use and attributes that you will want to consider before seeding your first crop.

GROWING CANNABIS

CHAPTER TWO

UNDERSTANDING THE PLANT

All of the benefits and side effects that we looked at in the previous chapter are dependent upon the particular strain of marijuana a person uses. Some strains will have stronger pain management effects, for example, while others will be more "heady" and relate to the effects that impact, or impair, the user's sense of perception. In this chapter, we'll see what exactly a strain is and how the genetics of our plants plays a role in determining the strain. There are two key categories within which most strains fall: sativa and indica. We'll explore what these descriptors mean and the rise of hybrid plants that combine traits from both types.

GROWING CANNABIS

Why Do Cannabis Genetics Matter?

We know how important genetics are when it comes to human beings. Our genes determine whether or not we are susceptible to certain illnesses, what we'll look like, and whether we'll be male or female when we're born. That last trait is determined by whether or not we have two X chromosomes (female) or an X and Y chromosome (male). The X chromosome in a human has around 800 different genes, while the Y chromosome contains only 70. The X chromosome contains about 150 MB of information while the Y chromosome has 3,300 MB. All of this data results in the amazing variety of human beings that the world sees today.

Cannabis is remarkably similar to humans in many regards when it comes to genetics. The plant has an X and a Y chromosome as well, though each chromosome contains between 800-850 MB of genetic information. Every single part of the plant, from how its leaves looks to the percentage of THC it has and even how it smells, is entirely determined by which genes the plant has. Growers work hard to breed plants together to isolate certain genetic traits they consider to be ideal. However, there are so many possible genes that cannabis can have that there is now a ton of research being done on creating a genetic map of cannabis. The goal of this genetic map is to allow researchers around the world to combine their data on traits and genes. With research moving in this direction, more and more designer strains will be popping up in the future.

When it comes to growing marijuana, genetics matter because they determine how the plant will grow, look, and affect the user. In the world of cannabis, plants come in male and female varieties just like humans. The female plant contains the bud, which is what people smoke. To create a hybrid plant, you take the male plant of one kind and have it fertilize the female of another kind. The seeds that the female plant produces now have traits from both types. The traits of the female plant will still be the strongest, but through multiple iterations you could grow a particularly effective strain that combines the best of both origin strains.

With that in mind, let's look a little more at what we mean when we talk about the various strains of cannabis.

What Are Strains?

GROWING CANNABIS

The cannabis plant began in Asia but then spread all throughout the world. One of the pieces of history that we saw in the last chapter was how the Vikings had acquired the plant and were able to get it to grow in their colder climate. In doing this, the Vikings essentially created their own strain of marijuana. Cultivators across the world have had to breed their plants to grow in a variety of different climates. As these plants grow, develop, and continue to mate and reproduce, they turn into what is known as strains.

Strains are essentially variations in the genetics from one cannabis plant to the next. Before, strains arose naturally because of the needs of the individual growers to acclimatize the plants. Today, however, with the advent of indoor gardening and the ability to control any plant's individual environment, strains have become much more about what genes a particular plant was grown to have. The global cannabis industry is expected to be worth more than $31 billion by 2021. This means that there is a lot of money involved in growing and where the money goes, skill follows. Skilled growers have now created thousands of strains of marijuana.

There are three general categories that strains fall into: indica, sativa, and hybrid. Each of these strains tells the user something about the effect that the strain will have when smoked (and we'll explore these each more in a moment). But within each of these categories, the various strains may have major differences, particularly when it comes to the compounds found in each strain. We looked at THC and CBD briefly but they are far from the only cannabinoids found in marijuana.

CBN helps in reducing the effects of neurological conditions such as epilepsy or seizures. THCA is similar to THC but is most useful in reducing inflammation and reducing neurological conditions associated with Parkinson's or ALS. CBG has been tied to reducing anxiety and other psychological issues such as OCD, PTSD, or depression. The proportion of these compounds present in the plant differs between strains.

Another area in which there is a wide variety is in the terpenes that are present and the quantity of them. Terpenes are a compound that naturally occurs in the plant and is primarily related to the way the plant smells. Marijuana is often described as flowery, skunky, or fruity in smell. Clearly, these descriptions would appear to be contradictory, since who ever heard of a fruit that smelled like a skunk. But it is the terpenes present in the strain that determines how the plant smells and creates this variety. It should be noted that while terpenes are most strongly associated with the smell, they also have effects on how the strain functions. A quick look at some of the most common terpenes will help enlighten this point.

Bisabolol is thought to help reduce inflammation and irritation of the body and has some microbial and pain-reducing effects as well. It also smells like chamomile. Limonene, on the other hand, smells like citrus and is thought to improve mood and reduce stress. Eucalyptol smells like eucalyptus, reduces inflammation, fights bacteria, and leaves the user feeling refreshed. Pinene smells like pine and helps ease nausea and pain. Linalool smells of flowers and helps boost mood. These are just a few of the many terpenes that are found in cannabis, each of which can be found in certain strains and may even help to give strains their names, such as Sour Diesel, which gets its name from its pungent aroma.

Let's take a look at a handful of strains. We cannot even begin to cover them all—that would easily take a book a dozen times the size of this one—but we'll look at some of the most common ones.

Sour diesel is known for its energizing and mood-lifting effects. Depending on the kind of work at hand, it can help provide a burst of productivity to the user's day and has been tied to the reduction of pain. Bubba Kush, on the other hand, helps relax the user and makes them sleepy. Hence, it is recommended to help fight insomnia. Bubba Kush is also linked to a reduction in pain and stress. A similar strain is Granddaddy Purple. Granddaddy Purple helps to induce sleep as well, but it also increases the user's appetite, which can be extremely useful for those whose medical issues result in a lack of appetite or nausea.

These strains are recommended for certain results because they have been grown to have the effects they do. Those mentioned above have been around for a while now, and this means that you can expect a certain level of consistency when using them. In contrast, newer strains or hybrids will show more variation between crops. Finding the strain that is right for you may take some time but sites like weedmaps.com and

GROWING CANNABIS

leafly.com compile information on the strains out there alongside what traits they have and even ratings from staff and users.

Figuring out what strain is right for you first starts by exploring the categories that were mentioned above: sativa, indica, and hybrid. Keep in mind, however, that individual strains of any one category may have effects that are not associated with that category. For example, indicas are seen as relaxing but a particular strain may in fact leave the user feeling more energized. The effects of marijuana should be viewed on a strain by strain basis, with the categories used to help the individual to narrow down their search for the right strain.

Sativa

GROWING CANNABIS

Sativas are known for the "heady" high that they provide when used. They tend to leave the user feeling invigorated. They're like the energy drink version of cannabis, only without all the sugar and dangerously high levels of vitamins. Many people find that sativas help them feel less anxious. They have also been linked to an increase in creativity in individuals, with people reporting that they feel they do some of their best creative work after using a sativa. Another link that has been seen is an increased ability to focus after using a sativa.

The sativa family comes from climates that are hot and dry. It prefers longer days, which means lights needs to be lit longer if growing indoors. Its origins are traced back to Africa, Central America, and Southeast and Western Asia, where the climate perfectly fits its needs. The plant itself tends to be tall but thin, with leaves that almost look like the fingers of a spread hand. They can pass twelve feet in height with the right conditions, but their height also means that they grow slower than other varieties. Because sativas are more of the "heady" experience, it is common for them to have high amounts of THC but low amounts of CBD.

Since sativas are stimulating, they are best used during the day as users may find it difficult to sleep after consumption. This makes the sativa most useful for individuals who work in the creative fields or who want to experience the psychological effects of cannabis over the physical benefits.

Indica

Indicas are most strongly associated with what is called a "body high." These strains are known for their relaxing properties and thus are among the most popular for battling insomnia, inflammation, nausea, and pain. A common use for indica is in reducing the side effects of chemotherapy. People undergoing chemotherapy often are so nauseated that they spend hours after each session vomiting. Use of an indica before a session has shown great results in reducing these side effects and helping patients keep their appetites and improve their mood.

Indicas find their origin from the plants of Afghanistan, India, Pakistan, and Turkey. In doing so, they are particularly well suited for growing in climates that are harsh or dry. They grow particularly well in the turbulent climate of the Hindu Kush mountains, after which many strains have been named (Purple Kush, Granddaddy Kush, Bubblegum Kush, the list goes on and on). Indica plants are much shorter than sativa plants. They tend to be short, stocky, and densely covered in bushy greenery. Whereas the leaves of the sativa are finger-like, the leaves on an indica are quite broad and more in line with what people think of when they picture a pot leaf. They grow much faster than sativa does, and they also tend to produce more buds, both of which make them a favorite amongst those who grow for financial reasons.

Indica is best consumed at night or when you are planning to stay at home and just relax. There is a common depiction of the cannabis user in the popular media as being too lazy to get off the couch. This image contrasts the effects of sativa but perfectly fits those of indica. The indica plant has much more CBD than the sativa and likewise also a lower ratio of THC, making it the more effective of the categories for medical purposes. However, this has begun to change due to the rise in hybrid strains in the last decade.

Hybrids

Hybrids are an interesting category of cannabis. They almost exclusively need to be created by growers, as the chances of a hybrid forming naturally in the wild is almost entirely impossible due to sativas and indicas preferring different climates. However, within a controlled growing operation, such climate variables can be accounted for to allow these disparate types of cannabis plants to interact with each other. Hybrids are formed by breeding an indica with sativa. Which category will be the stronger of the two depends on which is used to supply the female fruiting plant. The seeds produced are dominated by the genes of the female but with the genes from the other (male) brought into place. Because of this, hybrids have an especially large degree of variety as a category and even within an individual hybrid strain.

The appearance of a hybrid is entirely dependant upon the parent plants which were used to create it. The amount of THC or CBD they have is also dependant on this factor. However, hybrids are primarily created in order to increase the THC percentage of an indica or to increase the CBD percentage of a sativa, though the exact percentage of THC or CBD that a hybrid will have is a factor that cannot be accounted for in a generalization. This carries through to the effects most commonly associated with their use, as well as when they are best used.

GROWING CANNABIS

Ruderalis

Any discussion on cannabis plants would be remiss not to make a quick mention of the ruderalis. This kind of cannabis plant grows quickly and adapts well to extreme environments. They're small, rarely more than a foot tall, which makes them able to go from seed to harvest in roughly a month's time. They have almost no THC and only a little more CBD, though most likely neither is enough to produce effects in the user and so the plants are not used for recreational or medical purposes. However, the ruderalis is able to breed with sativa and indica plants. Their ability to breed across the board, along with their short growing time, make the ruderalis well suited for those individuals who want to experiment with creating hybrids, shorten the length of a strains growth cycle, or try to isolate particular genes for further use.

Chapter Summary

- The genetics of cannabis is shockingly similar to that of humans, even down to having male and female plants.

- The genes that a plant has are determined by the genes of its mother plant.

- The female cannabis plant is fertilized by the male plant and then produces seeds. The female plant is also the one to grow the bud which people smoke.

- Everything from the THC to CBD ratio to the smell of the plant is determined by the genes it has.

- Strains of cannabis are plants which share the same genes. Every strain has different genes and this allows for a wide variety of effects across thousands of strains.

- Strains can be divided into three general categories: sativa, indica, and hybrids.

- Other active ingredients in cannabis include the cannabinoids CBN, THCA, and CBG, all of which are found in different ratios depending on the genetics of the strain.

- CBN helps in reducing neurological effects such as epilepsy.

- THC reduces inflammation.

- CBG reduces anxiety and other psychological distressors.

- Many strains are named for the smell they have. Cannabis gets its smell from the terpenes which are present, another factor which is determined by genetics.

- Besides providing marijuana with its smell, terpenes may also have beneficial effects such as lifting mood or reducing inflammation.

- Experienced growers work hard to create powerful strains which provide the most beneficial effects possible.

- Older strains are more predictable, because they have had a long time of developing the same genetics from generation to generation. In contrast, newer strains may see a lot of variation between crops.

- While strains are split up into sativa and indica, a particular strain may actually have effects more commonly associated with the other kind, such as an indica that has the energizing effects of a sativa.

- Sativas are associated more with the "high" of marijuana, producing the most notable psychological effects.

- Sativas grow tall and slow, enjoying hot and dry climates with long days.

GROWING CANNABIS

- Sativas are high in THC but tend to have low CBD. They are best used during the day because of their energizing effect.

- Indicas provide the most body-heavy effects, such as reducing pain or inflammation.

- Indicas flourish in harsh climates. They are shorter, faster growing, and produce more buds than sativa plants.

- Indicas are known for their high CBD ratio and a subsequent lower amount of THC.

- Hybrids are combined by breeding a sativa with an indica. Their preferred climate, appearance and effect will be determined by the parent plants.

- Hybrids are often created to raise the THC level of indicas or the CBD level of a sativa.

- A hybrid will have the strongest genes from the mother plant, leading people to categorize hybrids as either sativa-indica or indica-sativa with the mother plant's type coming first.

- Hybrids have the most variety in the genes of their strains.

- There is also a class of cannabis plant called the ruderalis. This plant does not produce enough THC or CBD to have an effect when consumed, but it can mate with either sativas or indicas, which makes it useful for growers looking to isolate genes.

GROWING CANNABIS

- The ruderalis also grows the quickest of any type, from seed to harvest in roughly a month, which makes it ideal for combining with other plants to create quicker growth cycles.

In the next chapter, you will learn about the ways in which the growth of cannabis is affected by the environment it grows in. Cannabis is grown both indoors and outdoors, and you will see the pros and cons of both options in order to pick the optimal setup best for your specific needs.

CHAPTER THREE

WHERE TO GROW YOUR MARIJUANA

When it comes to gardening, there are two options available to us. We can either grow our crops outdoors and rely on the climate of where we live and the unpredictability of Mother Nature or we can design our crops to grow indoors, where we can control the climate and remove variability from the equation (if we are mindful and remove chances for infection or pests).

Cannabis is a particularly flexible plant, able to flourish both indoors and outdoors. Outdoor growers may choose to include a plant or two in their backyards among bushes or flower beds. They can also drop seeds throughout a forest and come back to find plants that survived to harvest. Of course, the primary method for outdoor growing is to plant a proper crop and oversee it through the growth cycle, which is what we'll be considering when we look at outdoor growing, but it is truly impressive just how versatile cannabis can be when it comes to growing.

GROWING CANNABIS

Indoor growing is the more popular approach these days. Growing indoors allows the gardener to control the conditions the plant experiences. This allows for the conditions to be set just right for the most plentiful harvest. It also allows the gardener to reduce contamination from the environment or accidental fertilization from another strain. However, growing indoors presents its own challenges which must be considered as well. Let's take a look at the key differences between these two approaches and then consider them each themselves.

Growing Indoors versus Outdoors

Making the decision on where to grow your cannabis requires that you consider three primary factors. The first factor is the amount of control you have over the growing process. While you may naturally assume that more control is always a good thing, you will see this isn't quite true. The next factor, and the only factor that matters to many people, is the upper limit you are willing to spend on growing. This cost factor goes hand in hand with control; the more control you want, the more you can expect it to cost you. The final factor is the quality of the cannabis. We aim for the highest quality, but getting there will be determined by the other two factors, your skill level, and your luck.

Growing your cannabis indoors allows you to take over full control of the growing process. Cannabis doesn't just grow inside the house by sitting in a pot in the corner or next to the window. The cannabis plant requires that you consider its needs and build an area dedicated to its growth. If properly laid out, then this area will allow you to control everything about the plant's environment from the temperature to the lighting to the CO_2 production to the humidity. It will also allow you to easily get around the plant for harvesting, trimming, and upkeep.

Growing indoors often provides the best product. However, the power of a light bulb is nothing compared to the power of the sun. Indoor plants will produce fewer buds, and the plants will not be as strong. There are other issues involved in creating an indoor growing environment that passes as natural. One issue that will come up when we look at pests is the way that growing outdoors actually leads to fewer problems with mites when compared to growing indoors. This can make outdoor farming sound like a good idea, but growing outside only works when you live in a climate with the right amount of heat, sun, and humidity.

You need to consider the cost of operations when making your choice. However, you are going to be spending a decent amount of money regardless of the option you pick. It may cost more to start growing indoors because you will need to purchase climate control systems, but once that is in place, the cost levels out a little more. Because an indoor grow operation has a high turnover, the grower will always have something they can do to help the plants out. This eats up a lot of time. But growing outside takes a lot of time to plant a crop, and then crop maintenance will require several hands. In addition, depending on the size of the crop, you may need to hire more hands when it is harvest time. This is because outdoor crops work by a seasonal basis and so everything is ready to harvest at the same time. The time and labor spent can quickly run up the cost of growing. If you are concerned about how much it will cost you to grow, it is a good idea to sit down ahead of making your decision and write out a budget and plan.

It is also a good idea to consider the way that each style of growing makes income. Indoor farming has a high startup cost but allows you to control the breeding of plants to make unique and high-end strains that are more potent. Indoor growing also harvests many times throughout the year, and so your income trickles in periodically. However, indoor growing also takes a lot of electrical energy since your lighting will replace the power of the sun. This cost in energy is subject to change, with almost every projection of the future saying that the price of energy will go up. An outdoor crop takes barely any energy at all and it produces much more buds. You might only be making an income on a seasonal basis, but the increase in yield means you may make more money off of it. However, the THC amount will typically be lower, and so it will not sell for as much as the indoor cannabis does.

Indoor growing leads to the best product. All of the highest quality strains are grown indoors, without fail. Having the ability to control the growing climate and speed up the breeding process has led to some amazing strains. Along with controlling the climate, you have the ability to control the CO_2 level in your growing area. Higher CO_2 levels lead to faster growth and higher THC levels. By remaining indoors, the plants aren't exposed to any harmful environmental factors like wind or rain that could harm them. The buds on your plants only risk one thing harming them: You. If you handle your plants properly, and prevent infection or infestation, then the plants shouldn't have any troubling degradation.

Where the indoor plants are completely under your control, the outdoor plants are under the control of Mother Nature. They typically don't look nearly as pretty as indoor plants do, with a product that isn't as appealing aesthetically, despite their chemical components being perfectly fine. There are many people who prefer the look of a natural, outdoor grown bud and so this may work to your advantage if you are crafty. There is an idea that outdoor grown cannabis is always ugly. This comes from the fact that many outdoor growers are doing so outside of the law, and so the plants and the yield are cared for quickly rather than carefully.

However, a change has slowly been impacting the market. With the legality of cannabis, there are now many farmers using greenhouse techniques to combine aspects of both indoor and outdoor growing. This is by far the most expensive option and it is yet to be seen if these growers will be able to stay afloat on the income it provides. Time will tell whether or not this technique should be explored in more depth. For now, let's turn our attention towards outdoor growing for a few moments.

GROWING CANNABIS

Growing Outdoors: The Best Places to Grow

The best part of growing outdoors is the many options available to you in terms of location. You could grow just about anywhere you can imagine. However, there are some locations that prove to be the most popular. There are also some concerns that should be addressed when picking your location, such as security.

Many, many different places have been used as grow sites over the course of human history (and especially as of recently), and this means that there are a lot of voices sharing their experiences. The best place that you can grow your cannabis is in your own garden. This gives you access to it whenever you want. However, if you have an open garden then it can be very easy for people to come and steal your product. This is unfortunately a more common problem for growers than you might imagine. More security is offered by growing on a balcony or on a roof terrace.

However, the visibility of these plants may not be appreciated by your neighbors, and strong or persistent wind can be damaging to the plants. Fields are great locations for growing sites because they are open to lots of sun, but they certainly make your harvest noticeable and this means a need for more security. Many growers who focus on smaller crops consider forests to be ideal locations. If it is off the beaten path and hence offers a much higher level of security, but it can be more difficult for plants to receive the proper amount of sunlight and water. Regardless of where the grow site is, being close to a river means the soil stays wet, and this can help your plants to stay properly hydrated.

Which of these locations is ideal depends on whether or not they are able to give your plants access to the environmental elements they need the most. Cannabis requires a lot of sunlight, with the various strains liking more or less on an individual basis. It also helps to have water nearby and to ensure that there is a breeze, but not one so powerful it can damage the plants. Soil that is rich in nutrients or that you can make rich yourself is almost (but not quite) a must. You also need to have easy access to continue caring for them throughout their growth. But one of the biggest issues is security. Thieves are common in this industry, and you do not want to lose out on some major money because you hadn't considered the threat they pose.

Even though growing outside means relying on the whims of nature, you are still able to take over control of some of the elements. For example, if you aren't able to find soil that is naturally rich, you can purchase your own. Or, if you aren't able to find a location close to water, you can set up a watering system to compensate. The primary elements that make a location ideal is how much sunlight it gets, how much wind it is exposed to, and whether or not you can keep the plants protected from outsiders.

Growing Outdoors: Growing Calendar

Because growing outdoors ties you to the changing seasons, it means there is a very specific schedule from which you will be operating. Cannabis requires a certain amount of illumination each day, or photoperiod, so it can move from the vegetative stage into the flowering one. The following calendar is based on what is best for growers located in the Northern Hemisphere.

The best time to germinate your seeds is at the start of April, but it can be done in April, May and June. It is recommended that you germinate your seeds indoors at this period prior to heading outdoors. Depending on when you first started the germination process, you will be ready to move your seeds to their outdoor location between May to July. You can expect to need to top the plants between June and the start of August. Pruning and clean up will take from August to September. Then, if everything previous has gone well, and there have been no major disasters, the harvest season begins halfway through September and can last as late as mid-November.

It should be noted that where you are located affects these dates, even within the Northern

Hemisphere. For example, Californian farmers will have a longer period to work since the weather is always so warm there. Those in Washington, on the other hand, will find that they have to wait until later in the season to germinate if they want their plants to receive enough sunlight to stay healthy and they'll even need to harvest earlier because the weather turns so drastically.

You can use the Spring and Fall Equinoxes, along with the Summer and Winter Solstices, to help provide a rule of thumb for when things should be done. The Spring Equinox is a good time to get your seeds ready. The Summer Solstice is all about the sun getting higher in the sky, and this means better weather for your plants, so make sure they're outside now. When the weather starts to get colder and the sun starts getting lower, you will notice that your plants have started to fruit. But hold off on harvesting until the Fall Equinox. Finally, remember to have everything harvested and dried in time for the Winter Solstice.

This provides a useful window for when to start working on what step. Just remember that this guide needs to be slightly adjusted in order to fit your local area. A warmer climate doesn't need to worry about starting off indoors, they can go straight outdoors. Harvesting, on the other hand, has to be done earlier in colder climates. Use a growing calendar to get a starting time frame and then examine your local environment to fine tune your plan.

GROWING CANNABIS

Growing Your Plants Indoors

When it comes to growing plants indoors, you have several options at hand for how you want to go about it. You could set up a tent in which to grow your plants, or you may even set aside an entire room to be your "grow room." Another popular way of growing indoors is to use what is called a grow box, which is just an enclosed system in which your plants grow. Each of these approaches can produce amazing results. However, regardless of the option you choose, there is still going to be a lot to set up when preparing to grow indoors. Understanding the eight steps necessary for growing indoors is the most effective way to cover everything you need and see if the process sounds like something you can handle.

The first step is to decide on the space that will be dedicated for the purposes of growing. As previously mentioned, this could be a closet, tent, grow box, room, or even just the corner of a room. When you are first starting out, it can be a good idea to start small. You are likely to make mistakes in the beginning and the smaller your setup, the less money is wasted on mistakes. You can also get a good sense of the growth cycle and how to care for plants best when you start small. Less plants means you can really take your time to watch and learn how they grow and evolve and see how often upkeep is demanded. However, keep in mind that you will likely want to expand your operation as time goes on. Picking a space which you can add more plants to is a great way to keep costs of expansion down.

You may have chosen to use a tent or a grow box for your designated area. These are smaller systems, so your way of tending to the plants will be to remove them from the growing area and work on them outside of their environment. You will need to have a space in which you can look after the plants while exposing them to the minimal amount of risk. Keep this in mind if you go with these smaller options; they do not take up a lot of space but you need to have some available for care. Tents and grow boxes are great because they are sealed against light, but you need to remember that your maintenance area has to be sealed as well. Your plants expect it to be dark at certain times and light at others. If light gets in when it is supposed to be dark, it may confuse the plants and detrimentally affect their growth.

Remember that your growing area is not just going to be filled with plants. You also need to have enough space for important equipment, such as lights. High quality lighting is the most important part of your operation. There are three kinds of lights that see the most use for cannabis growing.

High intensity discharge (HID) lights are the standard of the industry because they balance efficiency, value, and output. They will cost you more than the other types, but they shine bright as can be. You can get them in metal halide or high pressure sodium designs. Metal halide bulbs are great for vegetative growth while the high pressure sodium bulbs are most effective during the plant's flowering stage, and some growers opt for both designs to maximize efficiency.But if you can only afford one type of bulb, high pressure sodium bulbs are the better ones to use. HID lights will also need a ballast and a hood or reflector for each bulb used.

Fluorescent grow lights are very popular for growers that see cannabis gardening as a hobby. High output bulbs are the most popular fluorescent grow lights because they provide a good amount of light but do not require a cooling system like HID lights tend to. They also cost less when building your setup because they usually have everything you would need, such as reflectors or ballasts, in a kit for purchase. However, fluorescent grow lights produce around 25% less light per watt of electricity than the HID bulbs do. This means that you will typically need to use more fluorescent grow lights and this could easily crowd your grow space.

LED grow lights have started to be used more often because of how efficient they are, but as a downside, they can also cost upwards of ten times the amount of a HID system. But these lights last for long periods and use less electricity. This means that they also produce less heat, which may save you on the cost of cooling. They offer the widest spectrum of light outside of the sun, which means better yields.

Regardless of what lighting source you decided on, your plants are going to need some ventilation. Your plants need both fresh air and CO_2. You're going to want to have air flowing through the growing space for this reason. A typical setup for this is to have an exhaust fan near the top of your room with a filtered inlet close to the floor on the other side of the room. No matter how much air you have moving, you need to ensure that you stay within 70°F-85°F when the lights are on and 58°F-70°F when the lights are off. Because temperature is so important, you will likely find yourself matching your exhaust system to your plants' temperature needs. One way to figure this out is to turn your lights on for a few hours and then take the temperature. This allows you to see how much you have to control through your ventilation.

The next step, which most growers take but isn't a necessity, is to automate as many pieces of the system as possible. You can use timed switches to control the light/dark cycle or get a smart thermostat to monitor the space's temperature and control how the ventilation is running. This step is used to give you more free time, since most people cannot change their schedules to fit the needs of their plants.

Growing outdoors means that you typically rely on the growing medium provided for you. But when you grow indoors, you pick that medium ourselves. Soil is the most widely used medium because it allows the widest room for error. Another highly popular method is to use a hydroponic system, in which the plants take their nutrients from a liquid solution you have created to provide them with everything they need. A hydroponic setup is going to be much more expensive and detailed, but there are quite a few advantages that make hydroponics an impressive approach. While considering the medium, you should be considering what sort of pot or tray you will grow the plants in. Your medium may determine your container. For example, a deep water culture means your growing medium must be water.

No matter which medium you choose, the plants will want access to nutrients. Cannabis plants need nitrogen, phosphorus, and potassium, as well as calcium, magnesium, iron, and copper. Some growing mediums are fertilized for you. But if yours is not, then you will need to create a nutrient solution yourself. You can purchase nutrients in liquid or powder form and create your own water-based mix.

Finally, you are going to have to water your plants (unless you choose to use hydroponics). This means you will want to have easy access to your plants and have enough space for them to drain away. This takes up more space from your growing space. It is vitally important to have a proper drainage system in place, too, because stagnant water is unhealthy for your plants and can breed harmful viruses.

All together, growing indoors requires you to have enough space to properly tend your plants. A tent and grow box may allow you to keep the space small, but you still need to be able to take the plants out and tend for them properly, so leave yourself enough room to do so. Growing indoors comes with costs that the outdoors avoids but the control you have over your plants when growing indoors is unparalleled.

GROWING CANNABIS

Chapter Summary

- Where you grow your cannabis is ultimately a choice between indoors and outdoors: control or nature.

- Growing indoors will let you take control of the process and have total power over the grow environment.

- Growing indoors also tends to produce better quality product but in much smaller yields.

- Both growing indoors and growing outdoors can be surprisingly expensive depending on the size of your operation.

- Growing outdoors is dependent on a seasonal calendar while growing indoors allows you to artificially make the conditions the cannabis needs to grow.

- Higher CO_2 levels when growing indoors allows the cannabis to grow faster and with higher THC levels.

- You can grow just about anywhere outdoors so long as the plants get enough sun and aren't exposed to overly strong winds.

- Growing near a river or lake is great for giving the plants the moisture they crave.

GROWING CANNABIS

- When growing outside it is important to consider security as thieves are a real issue when farming cannabis.

- The growing calendar for outdoor crops can be divided into four sections: the Spring Equinox when you have your seeds ready; the Summer Solstice when your plants should be in the ground; the Fall Equinox for when you are harvesting; and the Winter Solstice by which everything should be dried.

- The first step to growing indoors is setting up a location that you can control, keep clean, have access to the plants and enough space for lights and equipment.

- HID lights are powerful but costly. Fluorescent grow lights are popular but create less light. LED grow lights are expensive but use less energy while also providing plenty of light.

In the next chapter, you will learn about cannabis seeds and how to differentiate between sativa, indica, ripe, and premature seeds. You will also learn how to germinate your seeds to prepare them for planting. Then, you will learn how to plant them and the lighting, temperature, and airflow your seeds need to grow, as well as how to care for your seedlings once they have sprouted.

CHAPTER FOUR

GERMINATION OF SEEDS

While growing marijuana focuses primarily on the bud that is produced, every plant begins with a seed and so shall we. In this chapter, we will contemplate how to pick our seeds, plant them, properly care for them, and see them through to the next stage in their growth. It is only from beginning with and properly nursing our seeds that we can achieve our desired results down the road.

Picking the Right Seeds for You

Cannabis seeds are only produced by female plants after pollination by a male plant. This is important to note because it tells us that the female plant is more valuable to us than the male plant because it can actually allow us to harvest our own seeds. We'll need to purchase or acquire seeds to begin with, but if we are attentive gardeners then we will be able to use our own seeds in the future. When we plant a regular seed, there is a 50/50 chance that the seed is male or female. However, only female plants produce the bud we want to harvest, so we are doubly interested in having more female plants. We can do this by purchasing seeds that have been feminized. This way we can ensure that we'll grow lots of female plants.

Just remember, we still want some male plants in order to fertilize our own females.

In order to feminize a seed, a seed is either sprayed with a solution of colloidal silver, treated with a method called rodelization, or sprayed with gibberellic acid. You can purchase seeds that have already gone through one of these processes and then use the process yourself with your own seeds down the road. These seeds will be almost identical to the female plant that parented them. This is otherwise known as cloning a plant, and we'll be looking at how that is done in the next two chapters.

When you are choosing which seeds to plant, there are a few factors that you can use to help you make your decision. The color of the seed is important. A

GROWING CANNABIS

healthy seed is dark in color, generally tan, brown, or black. Seeds that are lighter or even green should be avoided. Seeds will also have patterns on them that you can use to figure out if they are sativa or indica. Sativa seeds are typically a solid color while indica seeds have a striped pattern. You should also check how hard your seeds are. The harder the seed, the better it is. Do not even bother planting a soft seed; they are unlikely to produce a healthy plant.

Seeds come in various qualities, but the highest quality seeds are those that were harvested only after they were given a chance to fully mature. The environment the seeds are exposed to is also relevant, with the highest quality seeds being those that are stored in dark, dry places where they can cool off. If the seeds are allowed to mold, then they aren't going to be worth planting. Keep in mind the age of the seeds. If they have not been frozen, then they should be no older than sixteen months. If they have been frozen, then age becomes irrelevant. What really makes high quality seeds stand out from the rest is their genetics. Great genetics means high quality plants. Ask about the genetics of the seeds before you buy them. Find out what strains the parents were to see if they are compatible and make for desirable buds.

Finally, while all the talk about quality and care is important, the real answer to what seeds you should pick comes down to what you are looking to grow. Do you want to grow a sativa or indica or even a hybrid? Pick the right seed for what you want to grow. Make your choice based on strain and use these practices to weed out lower quality seeds so that you only plant the best.

Planting the Seeds

What we want to do when planting our seeds is provide everything they need to germinate. This is the process through which a seed becomes a plant. Marijuana seeds need water, heat, and air in order to properly germinate. While there are many techniques used to germinate seeds these days, the easiest is still the most common. You will want to have a couple of clean plates and a roll of paper towels at hand.

Soak four sheets of the paper towel in distilled water. You want them to soak, but you do not want them to leak water. Drain away any excess water before you set them down on the plates. Put two sheets onto each plate. Next, take your seeds and place them on the plates with about an inch of room between them. Once they are set out, use the other two sheets to cover them. You should have two plates of seeds sitting on soaked paper towel with wet towels covering them. You want to keep these seeds in a dark place where they will be protected from harm. One way to do this is to use another plate, flipped upside to create a lid. Store the plates somewhere between 70°F-90°F.

You're going to have to wait for nature to do its part now. Check on the plates from time to time to make sure that the paper towels are still wet. If you find they are drying up, then adding some more water will be beneficial for the seeds. Rewet the towels by sprinkling water on them or using a spray mister. Some

GROWING CANNABIS

seeds germinate quickly while others take some time, upwards of a few days even. You will know that a seed has germinated properly if it splits apart and a single sprout comes out. This sprout is called the tap root and it is the main body of the plant. As the plant grows, this root remains at its center. Keep in mind that you do not want to touch your seeds until they are ready to grow, as premature handling can cause issues in the splitting or the emergence of the tap root.

Once the seeds germinate, it is then time to plant them. Most growers transfer their seeds over to small pots initially. Doing this allows you to focus on the plants individually, making sure they grow strong enough to make it through to joining the main tray. Fill up your trays with a suitable potting soil, one that is breathable. Use a finger to make a small hole, about ¼ of an inch down. You will want to use tweezers or something similar to move the seed. It's important to be gentle now. Put the seed into the hole with the tap root down. Cover the hole and the seed back over with soil. Water the soil, starting with a spray bottle. You want to start with a spray to avoid drowning the seed. Keep an eye on the temperature of the pot to make sure it stays within the proper ranges below.

In five to seven days, you will notice a small seedling beginning to rise out of the pot. If you do not, there may be an issue with the temperature, the amount of water, or even the seed itself. Give it a couple more days before giving up on the seedling, as it may just be a late bloomer. Seeds all grow at different rates, some quick and some slow, and some just do not grow at all.

GROWING CANNABIS

Do not worry if you end up with a slow grower, it could still end up being one of your best harvests.

Lighting, Temperature, and Air

When you are dealing with seeds, it is important not to let them have any light. Once you have planted them in the soil, you still do not want to expose them to light yet. However, they still need to have the right temperature while they are growing into seedlings. The ideal condition for the seeds is between 68°F and 82°F. They also want a bedding that is moist, so you should be checking the soil at least once a day and giving it a spritz if it is too dry.

Turn on the lights once the seedlings start to emerge from the soil. The seedlings want to have at least 18 hours of light each day, so be prepared for your grow room to be illuminated pretty much at all times. In fact, you can actually allow the seedlings to have 24 hours of light at this point without harming their growth too much. They are going to need a more diverse lighting schedule once they grow past the seedling phase. Since you are unlikely to be there to watch this happen, it is a good idea to use an 18/6 hour light/dark setup, which mimics a natural day/night pattern.

You can use HPS or MH lights with your seedlings, but they are not needed. Seedlings do just fine under more cost-effective LED grow lights. However, if you already have another type of light, then you can use it. MH lighting is more effective for seedlings than HPS lighting, as seedlings prefer the cooler blue light found in MH bulbs compared to the warmer red light in HPS bulbs.

It should take between ten to fifteen days for your seedlings to reach the vegetative stage of their growth cycle. Of course, it is important to avoid overly high or low temperatures, either of which may result in the plants' stunted growth or deformation.

Though often overlooked at this stage, it is important to note that the seeds need to breathe. If they do not have sufficient access to oxygen, they will suffocate. This is one of the reasons you want to use a spray bottle to lightly mist the soil rather than pour water directly on the soil. If the soil is heavy or soggy, the seeds will be unable to breathe. When too wet, the soil becomes a suffocating pillow over the seeds. The seeds need both moisture and oxygen.

You should also be careful not to plant seeds too deeply. When seeds are too deep, the soil above them becomes a suffocating weight, and even if the seeds do not suffocate from the soil, they face an entirely different issue. The shell of the seed provides needed energy to the seedlings to help them dig into the soil and set their tap root. But if the seeds are buried too deep then the seeds will not have enough energy to break out of the soil. You will have a bunch of popped seeds suffocating and dying before they can even reach the top. Always keep the seeds a quarter inch deep, do not go any deeper.

GROWING CANNABIS

Caring for Your Seedlings

We've seen how our seeds need to mature, can be kept for sixteen months and more when frozen, and like the dark. Taking care of your seeds is mostly done by leaving them alone to look after themselves. But your seedlings, on the other hand, are going to need some tender loving care. Cannabis plants are most vulnerable during the seedling stage, as they are very small and easily stressed or damaged.

Seedlings are at risk of being eaten, damaged by the weather, drowned, or worse. They do not have any real strength yet, and so it is up to you to ensure they're protected. One way to protect them is to use a transparent plastic bottle. Cut the bottle in half and stick it in the soil, so that the seedling is in the middle of it. This setup protects the seedling from pests while still allowing light to shine through. Make sure you cut air slits into the bottle, as the seedlings still need oxygen.

You want to make sure that the soil is moist, but overwatering can be a costly mistake. Too much water, as previously touched on, can suffocate the plant. We start our seeds in small containers rather than large ones because there is less risk associated with suffocation or waiting. In addition, the roots of the seedling do not sufficiently fill a large container and hence cannot reach all the water and nutrients it needs. But plants in a small container are easily overwatered and end up damaged for it. This problem changes as the seedling continues to grow. It will eventually get to a point where it's root system is too large for the small container. When this happens, you will have to move it to a larger container, or the root system will tangle and trap water in the container.

But just as overwatering can be a problem, underwatering your seedlings is also a problem. The roots of the seedling need to have access to plenty of water at all times. A lack of water will result in the plant wilting and the leaves staying too small or frail. If the soil in the pot is separated from the walls of the container then the environment is too dry for the seedling and you need to water it immediately. Plants that are grown in enriched soil risk growing strangely when they haven't been watered. They take on a dark shade of green and start developing growths in the wrong places. If you notice this, then you need to water the plants properly to save them. Check your plants every day to ensure that they have enough water.

Your seedlings will want to be fed nutrients. But you need to be careful not to create a toxic environment through overfeeding. When soil has too many nutrients in it, we call it "hot soil." This is because the plants will start to appear as if they have been burned. The tips of the leaves will be discolored, and you will need to water them with distilled water, which has had no extra nutrients or minerals added to it. But even if you have faced a toxic environment, they are still going to want to be fed. Now, however, you will need to be particularly wary about the nutrients you give to the plants. A good rule of thumb is to begin giving the seedlings a half dose compared to what you had been giving them prior to the hot soil issue. You can continue to increase the nutrient dose back to the package recommended dosage so long as you watch for issues.

The flipside of the hot soil issue is a lack of nutrients. If your plants are starving to death then you will notice that the leaves begin to grow all folded up. If you see folded leaves then you are going to want to add some nutrients to their mix. You may also want to check the pH level of the soil to ensure the soil is in a healthy range while growing. If the soil pH is outside of the optimal growing conditions, then the problem is that the nutrients in the soil aren't being absorbed properly. If you do not water them properly then they also will not be able to get the nutrients they need.

If you follow these steps and take care of your seedlings then you are well on your way towards your first harvest.

GROWING CANNABIS

GROWING CANNABIS

Chapter Summary

- Only the female plant produces seeds and only then after being pollinated by a male plant.

- The female plant is also the only one that produces bud, and so it is by far the most valuable of the plants.

- You can feminize cannabis seeds so that they sprout as females, where planting regular seeds gives you a 50/50 chance of getting a male or female plant.

- A healthy seed should be dark in color. Light colored seeds are premature. A healthy seed is also hard while a premature one is soft.

- Higher quality seeds are stored in dark and dry places.

- We need to first germinate our seeds, which can be done simply with a wet paper towel press.

- You will know that a seed is ready to move into the soil when the shell cracks and a tap root has emerged.

- Seeds should only be planted ¼ of an inch into the soil and then sprayed with water.

- While in the seed phase, these plants want no light.

- After five to seven days in the pot, a seedling should be seen emerging from the soil.

GROWING CANNABIS

- Seedlings like having 18 hours of light, a temperature between 68°F and 82°F and plenty of airflow.

- Overwatering seeds can kill them because the soil becomes too heavy and tight for oxygen to get through.

- Seedlings are small plants and can easily be harmed. Be very careful when doing anything with them.

- Underwatering your seedlings can cause they to wilt and look frail.

- Seedlings will be started on a nutrient diet but it is important not to overfeed them and create a toxin environment. If this happens then the environment will need to be rinsed with distilled water.

- An environment without enough nutrients will also harm seedlings. You can tell this is happening if the leaves of the seedling come in folded up.

In the next chapter, you will learn what a mother plant is and why it is so important when it comes to cloning plants. You will learn everything you need to know about picking the mother plant that is right for you and how to grow one that you can use again and again.

CHAPTER FIVE

WHAT IS A MOTHER PLANT?

When you find a strain that you absolutely love, you will want to use it repeatedly. The best way to make this happen is to keep around a mother plant, which is a plant that you keep in order to clone. Mother plants are kept in the vegetative state and aren't allowed to move into the flowering stage. Having a mother plant allows you to speed up the time needed for cultivation because you can simply clone the plant instead of repeatedly growing a new one from seed.

Keeping a mother plant on hand is highly efficient because it can reduce the time between cloning and harvesting to mere days. Choosing to clone instead of growing a daughter plant also minimizes any crop variations by ensuring that the characteristics of the strain stay consistent between plants and that every clone is a female. In this chapter, we'll see how to choose, grow, and maintain a healthy mother plant. The chapter after that will focus on how we use mother plants to clone plants.

GROWING CANNABIS

Choosing a Mother Plant

Mother plants are important to growers. Your mother plant is the source of much of the marijuana you grow, and it is the method through which you ensure that you are producing high quality buds on a consistent basis. Your mother plant is special, the creme of the crop. So it is important that you pick the perfect plant. The plant you pick is going to depend on what you enjoy. If you enjoy indica-type strains, then you aren't going to be growing a sativa mother plant. But regardless of personal preference, there are some tricks that you can use to ensure your mother plant is among the best of the best.

Nowadays there are many styles of feminized and autoflowering seeds available on the market. With feminized seeds you know you are guaranteed a female plant, which seems like a good fit for your mother plant. But most growers will tell you that you should only use normal seeds for growing your mother plant. Feminized plants have a higher risk of hermaphroditism. Your mother plant will be trimmed a lot to make clones, and this practice stresses the plant. When a feminized plant undergoes a lot of stress, there is an increased likelihood that the plant will flip its gender and start to grow male flowers. If such a phenomenon occurs, you will have to start all over. It is better to plant regular seeds and find a female the traditional way.

It is generally agreed that working with F1 hybrids is the best way to go about picking mother plants. An F1 hybrid is the first generation child of a cross between parents of two different strains. Your mother plant should be (though it doesn't have to be) one that you bred yourself by crossing strains. F1 plants tend to have the best aspects of their parents, and this means they have great genetics. F1 plants are also pretty quick growing compared to other seedlings, and this is great for maximizing your yield:growth ratio. You may also want to use an F2 hybrid, which comes from crossing two F1 hybrids. These plants are also amazingly potent, but on the downside, they take a lot of time to breed because you need to grow four plants, breed them twice, then grow two plants and breed them once. A single F2 hybrid requires six plants and three crosses. You can always work with regular seeds, but F1 or F2 plants will be the most impressive ones to turn into mothers.

GROWING CANNABIS

Since we use regular seeds rather than feminized ones, we will have to take the time to germinate them first. Grow the seeds as you would any other cannabis seeds until they reach the vegetative state. Then, starting three weeks into the vegetative stage, take some cuttings from them. This should be done early enough that the plants are still pre-flowering but late enough that the cuttings can take root. You want to take pre-flowering cuttings because the clones will be the same age as the cuttings. If your plants have already flowered, then your cuttings will as well. Take some time and label your cuttings so that you know which plants they came from. You will want to keep growing these cuttings like you did any normal plant, just remember to keep them labeled and to keep them separate from the original ones. Once your original plants flower, take note of their gender and remove any males as soon as you spot them. Head over to the clones you were growing (the cuttings) and remove the males from this group as well. This step is done to prevent them from pollinating a female before you are ready for such.

With the original plants flowering, keep your eyes on how they grow. If you are working with hybrids, then you will especially notice the way that each plant has its own unique features depending on which genes it received from its parents. You want to ensure that you turn the best plant into the mother plant. Which plant is the best will be up to you, but there are some markers that can help you decide.

Look at how vigorous the plants are. Since your mother plant will be trimmed often, you need a vigorous plant able to withstand the stress of cutting. Another trait that growers look for is the physical appearance of the plant. Some might prefer to smaller plants to save room, while others are partial to bigger plants. Coloring, spacing, and leaf size are all features that you may consider importance as well, depending on your taste. Yield is also a determining factor. You may want huge harvests, regardless of quality, or you may want smaller harvests of high quality. It's up to you. Also, use your nose and smell the plants. This may be a deciding factor in which you pick as your mother plant.

Growing a Mother Plant

Start with seeds and grow them through until they are in the vegetative growth stage and you can see what sex they are. Identify all of the females and take clones from them. You are going to want to take several clones from each female and then label which they came from for later reference. Continue to grow the new clones through to the flowering stage. You are going to keep the original plants in the vegetative stage. Remember that marijuana plants naturally react to the changing of the seasons and begin to flower when the days get shorter. To keep it in the vegetative growth stage is as simple as leaving the lights on it for 18 hours a day. Doing so tricks the plant into thinking it still isn't time to flower yet.

Your newly cloned plants will travel through to harvesting, and you should take the time to really examine how the yield turned out, the smell, the flavor, and everything else. When you have found the best plant, use that for your mother plant. Determine the mother of your preferred clone, and use that one as the overall mother plant.

A lot of growers like to offer extra protection to their mother plants by first growing them in an organic base. This is done so that the mother plants have the immunity necessary to fight off disease and stay strong. You will also want to be sure to use the original plant as your mother plant and not the clone that came from it. Plants that have been grown from a seed will have much stronger roots and immune systems.

It is worth considering the use of a nutrient solution specifically designed for mother plants. These mixes have nutrients to keep strong clones and healthy mothers. You really want your mother plant to have strong cell walls and high carbohydrate levels. Using too many nitrogen-rich nutrients is not good for mother plants, as doing so can lead to thin cell walls and low carbohydrates. Nutrients with a lot of calcium will help to improve both of these.

Mother plants will eventually start offering worse and worse clones. They'll grow much less vigilantly, while producing worse marijuana. If you are careful and take care of your mother plant, you can get a couple years out of it. But when the plant starts to offer diminishing returns, then you know that it is time to start considering what your next mother plant will be.

Chapter Summary

- A mother plant is a plant that is kept in the vegetative state to be used for cloning purposes.

- Your mother plant will likely be the best strain you can grow.

- You can use feminized seeds to get a mother plant but it is better to grow your mother plant from natural seeds instead.

- F1 hybrids are widely considered to be the best plants for use as mother plants.

- When your mother plant enters the vegative period you will take cuttings from it and grow these as cloned plants.

- You want your mother plant to be vigorous so that it can withstand the stress of all the cuttings you take from it.

- Take several clones from each potential mother plant you are growing so you can see multiple examples of how well it clones.

- Newly cloned plants will take less time to reach harvesting than those you grow from seed.

- Growers like to use an organic base when raising a mother plant so they gain immunities needed to stay strong.

GROWING CANNABIS

- Nutrient solutions are also powerful tools in helping mother plants stay healthy.

- Mother plants will eventually start to create weak clones, remember they do not last forever.

In the next chapter, we will continue our discussion of mother plants by looking at how you go about cloning your plants. We will cover the benefits of cloning plants to better understand why it is widely popular with both professional and hobby growers alike. You will then learn how to clone your own plants, which involves making more mother plants as well. We will also go over some of the mistakes that new growers make when they first start out, so that you do not fall into the same traps that others have.

CHAPTER SIX

CLONING YOUR PLANTS

We talked about cloning a lot in the last chapter because we actually have to first clone several potential plants to decide which should be our mother plant. It's easy to see how mother plants are intimately involved in the cloning process, but what we haven't touched on yet is the many reasons why you would want to clone a plant in the first place as opposed to just germinating and growing from a seed. First we'll tackle why you would want to clone a plant, then follow this with a detailed look at how you clone a plant. Combined with Chapter 5, this chapter will equip you with all the knowledge you need to choose your mother plant and clone your first plants.

GROWING CANNABIS

Benefits of Cloning Cannabis Plants

We spoke earlier about how you need to fertilize a female plant with a male plant in order to create seeds. These seeds then allow for the growing of new plants and this new plant will have features from both of its parents. This is the most classical form of breeding that there is. But it there is another newer way to breed a new plant through cloning. Cloning is a form of asexual reproduction because it does not require a male plant. To clone a plant is to take a cutting from it that will then grow into a new cannabis plant that is identical on a genetic level to the plant it was taken from.

Cannabis cultivation via cloning has taken off both on the industrial level as well as at the home grower level. This is because cloning offers many benefits that cannot be found through traditional breeding practices. Cloning a plant can save money, as you already have the materials necessary, and you do not need to go through the seedling phase that eats up so much energy. But that is only the most basic of the benefits that cloning offers.

If you grow an amazing plant that has high quality buds, you naturally want to grow more of that kind. Traditional breeding would mean that you have to combine two plants's genetics together. This would give you a third plant with genetics taken from its parents. It might produce buds of a similarly high quality, or it may grow buds of a lesser quality. That is the inherent risk of traditional breeding. But if you clone your plants, then you end up with an exact replica of your original plants with the same high quality buds. This means that you can keep growing the best stuff for quite some time to come.

Cloning is also useful if you want to isolate and replicate particular features. If you have a plant that grows quickly, then cloning it will allow you to produce many quick-growing plants. Or, if you have a plant with a flavor you really enjoy, then you can clone a bunch of these. If you have a higher number of plants on hand with your ideal features, you can experiment more and mate them the traditional way and see what kinds of plants you can come up with. This makes cloning particularly great for those who really enjoy getting deep with their crops.

Another great feature is the fact that cloning can basically give you a garden that is never empty. By skipping the earlier stages of the plant, you are able to shorten the time it takes to go from seed to harvest by only going from vegetation to harvest. While you will find that your clones get worse over time and you will need to replace your mother plant, you can get a lot of mileage out of cloning your plants. What's even better is that cloning isn't very hard at all.

How to Clone a Plant

First things first, you are going to need to grab a few things before cloning your plants. You will want to get something to cut the plants with. While many people reach for scissors, they actually aren't a great choice. Scissors often crush the branches they are trying to cut through, which can make it harder for the plant to take root. Instead, a razor that cuts but doesn't crush is a more professional choice. You will also want some water and the rooting medium and hormone that you will be using.

The best plants to clone are the mothers that are healthy and sturdy. They should be a couple months into the vegetative cycle as well. You can clone a plant as early as the third week of the vegetative period, but the clone will have a much better shot at rooting properly if you wait a little later.

You shouldn't just grab your razor blade and start hacking away at the mother plant. There are actually some steps you will want to take in the days before cutting. These steps will help to ensure that the mother plant receives as little shock as possible so that it can stay healthy and continue giving you clones for many harvests yet.

The first step you will want to take is to stop fertilizing the plant ahead of the cutting. The fertilizer

GROWING CANNABIS

has nitrogen in it, and while the plant needs nitrogen, it is better to allow time for the excess nitrogen to work its way out of the leaves before cutting. The reason you do this is to make it easier for the clones to take root. Excess nitrogen in the leaves and stem of the plant would signal the clones to try to grow vegetation when you want it instead to grow a root.

Remember to keep the work area sterile. This is where it becomes extremely important to have a proper location set aside for working on the plants if you are using a tent or grow box as opposed to a grow room. The environment should be sterile so that the freshly wounded mother plants and the cuttings you take do not become infected. A sick plant isn't a happy plant, after all.

It is time to start cutting. But first, you should determine the branches you want to cut. It is best to start at the lower branches which are generally the sturdiest and healthiest. You should be taking cuttings that are about 8-10 inches long. These cuttings should also each have several nodes on them. Once you have picked out the sections you want to cut, you will want to cut as closely to the main stem as you can. Your razor should be held at about a 45 degree angle to the branch. This is done to increase the surface area of the rooting space. A larger surface area means faster growth.

Now you should be holding a cutting in your hand. You want to immediately throw that into the water that you prepared at the beginning of the process. The water will prevent air bubbles from forming in the stem. These bubbles are deadly because they prevent the stem from absorbing water. An air bubble in the stem of your cannabis plant is pretty much as deadly as an air bubble in your bloodstream, and it can quickly kill a cutting. There are a lot of growers who cut along the stem of the cuttings even more at this stage as it purportedly helps to increase the rooting potential of the clone. It is a good idea to take the time to do this yourself so long as you do it prior to putting the cutting into the water.

With several clippings taken from your mother plants and moved over to water to keep safe, it is a good idea to clip their leaves. This helps the new clones have a more sanitary environment for when they root. It also helps the clones to make use of the processes of photosynthesis in a healthier manner. Use your razor, or even scissors on this part, and clip the fan leaves from the top down to about halfway down the stem. If there are any leaves near the bottom of the stem then you can remove these entirely so that none are left to just lay against the growing medium. Taking care of the leaves at this stage helps the clones to make better use of water and nutrients while rooting.

If you are working with rooting hormone, then this is a good time to drop the stems into your solution. Rooting hormone comes in gels, powders, and liquid solutions that have been formulated to help promote rooting and growth. You only need to dip the stem into the solution for a moment before you plant the clones into their new home. That home should either be Rockwool cubes, which allow for excellent airflow and hold moisture in well, soil, or straight water, if you are running a hydroponic setup. Each of these options have their strengths and weaknesses, so choose the one that is most appropriate for you and your grow space. You will be lighting these clones as if they were seedlings and providing at least 18 hours of light. You can purchase automatic tools, called auto-cloners, which take care of the water, oxygen, and light needs of the clones but these are quite expensive. For your first clones, I recommend taking care of the plant's needs yourself so you can get a proper feel for what goes into cloning.

The final step in cloning is the transfer back into the garden's circulation pots. You can tell that a clone is ready to be moved when you start to spot new vegetative growth beyond what it was planted with. Remember to be careful in moving the plant as it is still weak and you do not want to give it transplant shock, a common problem with cloning that arises due to overexertion of the plant and poor sanitation prior to transplantation.

Now you can sit back, watch your clones grow, and prepare for harvest. Once you have your seedling trays empty again, you can go ahead and start looking towards the next clones you want to prepare. Your mother plants will stay lit and stuck in the vegetative stage while your clones grow up, harvest, and earn you income. It should be a decent haul if you stick with cloning your most impressive strains!

GROWING CANNABIS

Mistakes New Growers Make When Cloning

We'll be looking at more mistakes that new growers make when it comes to cultivating marijuana, but here we are going to speak specifically about the most common mistakes that happen during the cloning phase. These simple tricks can help you to avoid a lot of pain and wasted time.

We've talked about it before but it has to be mentioned again: You must, absolutely must, keep your working area clean and sanitary. Use isopropyl alcohol to wipe down all of the surfaces that you will be working on. It is even a good idea to wipe down the surfaces around where you are working just in case you set something on them without thinking about it. A single mold spore can rain havoc on all of your cuttings. It is also a good idea to get single-use razor blades so that you never use an old razor for a new cut.

Cut everything you need to for this batch of clones then dispose of the razor and use a new one next time you are ready to do some cloning.

There are all sorts of rooting hormones out there on the market these days. But not all of them are worth their price. Many of them are downright awful. It is always a good idea to look at the reviews and see what people are saying about them. One of the best out there is Dip-n-Gro, which is used by professional arborists and cannabis cultivators the world over. Speaking of roots, there is a ton of writing on what is the best temperature for your roots. They have found that the best temperature to speed along new root growth is 78°F. There are many ways to achieve this heat, but one easy answer is to use a seedling heating mat. Just remember to get a thermostat that can be stuck into the growing medium. While we're talking mediums, you should use the same medium for your seedlings that you do your main crop.

Some people seem to think that clones need 100% humidity. There are actually some downsides to this. When you leave the humidity up that high you are allowing mold and wilt a window in which to grow. One idea to get around this is to use a humidity dome on your new clones for a couple days but make sure to get ones that have holes in them. The holes allow vapor to pass through and leave, which brings the humidity down lower while still providing help to your clones. The best part is that those vents make it nearly impossible for those pesky pathogens to grow.

If you are using a canopy, then you should consider the temperature it is at. 86°F is great for maximizing carbon dioxide uptake. However, it can be hard to keep this temperature since the rooting zone needs to be around 78°F. If you can get the canopy anywhere between those two numbers then that's awesome. The root zone temperature is more important than the canopy temperature but that doesn't mean you should just completely ignore the latter.

You can take some serious control of your lighting to really help out your new little clones. They need at least 18 hours of light, so plan to give them 18 hours of light and 6 hours of darkness. The best lighting for helping the roots to take hold is 120-200 umol m-2 s-1. If you are using T8 or T5 bulbs, then this shouldn't be any problem. As the roots start to take hold and grow, you can turn up the intensity by simply bringing the light closer to the plants and double checking the intensity. It can be useful to get yourself a PAR meter to be able to measure the light. In fact, you should just get one in general because there are all sorts of times that a PAR meter earns its weight in gold when dealing with your indoor cannabis operation.

Another mistake that is often made is to start your cloning with clones. The problem here is that when you use another clone that isn't quite mature, you are put in a spot where you will not really be able to predict how the plant's yield will turn out quantity or quality wise. If that plant turns out to be of poor quality then so will the rest of the clones you have growing. It is always better to start from a seed and work your way out from there. That way, you know what you are getting involved with.

GROWING CANNABIS

Many new growers will set themselves up with a mother plant that they absolutely love. It produces high-quality product or has the traits that they enjoy the most. So of course they will clone it like crazy. But the more this happens, the more they'll notice that later generations of clones aren't of the same quality they fell in love with. The THC and CBD levels degrade in time, and same with other elements such as smell, color, and sturdiness. Pay attention to the health of your mother plant and prepare to change it regularly, depending on how often you are cloning it. Most professionals advise changing mother plants after the fourth generation of clones.

A major issue is forgetting the water when cutting. You should either have water nearby to put the trimmings in or you should make your root cuts under running water. Either of these options work, the key is having that water to destroy any air bubbles in place. The problem with forgetting the water is that you will not immediately realize that an air bubble is killing your plant. The plant will get sick and slowly die, rather than just die off immediately. Because of this, you may find yourself checking the soil and nutrient solution when the problem was simply that you forgot to clear the trimmings before potting them.

Hopefully these simple tricks give you the advantage you need to be cloning amazing plants in no time.

GROWING CANNABIS

Chapter Summary

- To get seeds you need to have a male plant fertilize a female plant. This means that seeds will always require the genetics of two plants and that means a variety in the genetics.

- A cloned plant will always have the same genetics as the mother plant it came from and this means an identical plant, one that you know exactly what it provides.

- The predictability of cloning means the practice is very popular at all levels of the industry.

- Cloning can save money and allow growers to get more yield and income off of their best strains.

- The seeding phase of growing a plant uses a lot of energy. Cloning a plant can help you to save money by skipping this phase entirely.

- Cloning is great for isolating and replicating features that you want to continue breeding into further plants.

- Since cloning a plant can be done any time of the year, this can leave you with a garden that always seems ready to harvest.

- To clone a plant you want to select healthy mother plants that can survive the cutting process.

- Always stop fertilizing your mother plants before you take cuttings, as this prevents excess nitrogen from slowing down the clones' rooting process.

- It is important to keep the work area sterile to avoid infection. Always wipe and clean anywhere you plan to work and the surrounding areas that you might accidentally touch.

- You want your cuttings to come from the lower branches that are around 8 to 10 inches from the bottom, and these cuttings should have multiple nodes on them.

- Use your razor to cut at a 45 degree angle on the branch so that there is a larger rooting space for your clones.

- Next you are going to want to put the cuttings into water to get rid of air bubbles. Air bubbles left in a clone will kill it slowly and leave you wondering what the problem was.

- Clip the leaves of the cuttings so that they can more easily use photosynthesis.

- Drop the cuttings into rooting hormone. You will also want to cut at the roots a little to create a more direct connection between the root and the soil.

- Plant the cuttings and you got yourself a clone.

- New growers often forget to keep the work area sanitary and this leads to deadly results.

GROWING CANNABIS

- Experiment with rooting hormones to find the one that works best for you. Cheap hormones get poor results.

- Too high of humidity risks mold and wilt, clones should have high humidity but be allowed to breathe.

- Keep the temperature of the rooting zone around 78°F.

- The new clones will want at least 18 hours of light.

- Do not start cloning from clones, always clone from a plant grown out of seed.

- Remember that mother plants degrade, plan to replace it after three generations.

- Never forget the water when cutting, it is necessary to keep your plants alive and well after all.

In the next chapter, you will learn how to finally harvest your crop. You will first learn how to tell that your marijuana is ready for harvest by examining the color of the trichomes. Then you will learn a step-by-step process for how to harvest your plants yourself. This guide will go over how to prepare your workspace, flush your plants to prevent contamination, physically harvest the plants, and then trim them to look beautiful and appeal to buyers.

CHAPTER SEVEN

HARVESTING YOUR CROP

For many, harvesting is the most exciting part of the whole process. Who can blame them? If you consume marijuana then this is what you were building up for and now you get to enjoy the fruits of your labors. And if you are growing for money, well, now you get to make that income.

If you are growing outdoors then it has taken a long time, too. You've had to wait as it matured and grew. But is it fully grown, just because it is within that window specified in Chapter 3? Before you go ahead and harvest, it is always a good idea to take a deeper look at your plants to make sure they are ready. We'll see in this chapter how to determine the readiness of our crop, as well as harvest our cannabis, and learn about trimming it.

How to Tell If Your Marijuana Is Ready for Harvest

GROWING CANNABIS

The window of harvesting is going to be set by the strain type rather than by the calendar we saw earlier. The calendar is a good guideline for the basic steps of when the harvesting opportunity is available, but it is always best to check your plants and respond to what they are telling you. While they do not have mouths from which to tell us how they are feeling, the cannabis plant has many ways of announcing that it is ready to harvest. This is important because when you harvest is more important than you may think.

Marijuana is primarily used to get high, and that makes the effects of the plant very important in regards to determining its value. The high will first be affected by the strain, and as you already know, different strains have different effects. Sativa strains have different effects from indica ones, and then even within a type there is a lot of range. Each strain has additional variety to it, as told by descriptors such as bubba, skunk, kush, haze, and purple. All of these words (and more) are used to describe a variation of the strain itself, and you will see these variations pop up across many strains, all to let the purchaser know what to expect. Finally, the most important in terms of harvesting is the amount of time that has gone by between the start of the flowering stage and the harvest. The amount of THC glands that have been allowed to develop is determined by how much time the plant has had to flower. The longer the time it has had, the more mature the plant is considered to be and the more THC it will have.

When you look at a marijuana bud up close you see leafy plant matter, little hairs, and numerous specks of white crystal. It is these crystals that hold all of the

THC. In the cannabis community, this part is simply referred to as the crystal. However, they are really called trichomes. It takes a few weeks of flowering for trichomes to form, but they quickly start to multiple, grow, and mature once they initially form. These trichomes tell us how much THC the marijuana will have, and they also serve as the best guideline for deciding if your plants are ready to harvest because they help us estimate the plant's maturity at a glance through their color.

There are four trichome colors to understand. The first is translucent, in which the trichomes appear like little water droplets on the bud. This tells us that the plants are not fully matured yet. Essentially, these plants have very little THC, and nobody is going to purchase or use this marijuana if you harvested it now. Such a plant would also have a much smaller yield, since much of it would be unusable. On the other hand, if the trichomes are amber, then the plants are overly ripe. These plants, however, are still sellable, as overripe trichomes are linked to a "body high."

GROWING CANNABIS

The majority of growers harvest their plants when the trichomes are a cloudy color. They still look like little water droplets on the bud, but you cannot see through them anymore. At this stage, the bud is at its ripest and most potent stage. However, some people like to wait just a little bit past this stage. As the trichomes start to become overripe and just take on an amber color, you can harvest them to get a combined effect in which the high is shared between the mind and the body. This makes for a widely enjoyed type of high that many people think is the best.

Indica strains can be expected to mature far quicker than sativa ones. Between six to eight weeks after flowering, you should be harvesting. Start examining the trichomes around week five to find the best window in which to harvest. Meanwhile, sativa strains will take between eight and twelve weeks to mature. In fact, sativa plants may take even more depending on the particular strain. To be safe, you should start checking the trichomes around week eight of flowering.

The best way to check on the trichomes is to put a bud underneath the microscope. Most photos of marijuana made the trichomes look huge, but they are really quite small and hard to see with the naked eye. Pretty much any pocket scope will give you enough magnification to see them clearly. You should expect the trichomes to be clear when you first look, then you want to keep checking them daily to watch as they shift. It is up to you whether you want to harvest for a head high, a body high, or a combined head and body high. It all depends on your goal with that particular yield. Remember to wear gloves and handle the plants carefully. You would hate to damage them now when they're this close to ready.

There are a couple other indicators that let you know it is harvest time. The trichome is merely the most popular and widely used method. You can also look at the color of the little hairs on the bud. These are called pistils or stigmas. Immature plants will have yellow-white pistils. By the time the plant is mature, they will be orange. There are also the swollen calyxes, which are little pods on the bud. These indicate if a plant has been pollinated, as they will have seeds in them if so. But in unpollinated plants, the swollen calyxes slowly swells throughout the flowering period as well. When they are nice, thick, and plump, the plant is signalling you that it is ready to harvest. You can also determine how mature the plant is by the overall size of the buds. They will continue to grow until they begin to slow and eventually stop. Growing buds are not the best sign for judging maturity, but it certainly can be considered when taken along side the other pieces we've looked at.

So if your plants are nice and mature, it's time to harvest!

A Step-By-Step Guide to Harvesting Your Plants: Preparation

The first step, before you pull the first bud off the plant, is to get everything prepared and ready for the harvest itself. You are going to want to set aside enough space for all of your plants. It is a good idea to handle them all in the same place, because otherwise the odor can get everywhere. Marijuana has a strong smell, and when you have an entire crop's worth, it gets especially smelly.

But you also want to set aside a designated location so that you can control the temperature of the room. You're going to want to keep it at 70°F or below. This is to stop the cannabis oils from volatilizing, which again will help to reduce the odor. If the room is too hot, then they are going to really start stinking up the place. It can be a good idea to seal the room and then install a vent, but this is only for really large harvests.

You're going to need some tools to handle this. First off, gloves are going to be a must. You will want them to be latex or nitrile. These will help to stop the buds from getting contaminated. They will also help to keep your hands clean when handling the fresh buds as the buds can be extremely sticky. You will also want to get trimmers, which could be scissors or electric trimmers designed for the job. Whichever you go with, you will be using them a lot, so a trimmer tray is also a good idea. Trays make it easier to sort the harvest and excess product, crystal or kief, can be caught in the trays so you do not lose anything when working through it. You will probably also want to set up some lines throughout the room that you can hang the bud from. These will help you to dry out the product.

With the tools prepared, it is time to prepare the plant next. The first step is to remove old leaves. These are the leaves lowest to the ground. You will notice that they have turned, or are starting to turn, yellow rather than green like the rest of the plant. These leaves are stealing energy away from the buds. However, it is important to only trim when you are preparing for the harvest. It is also important to keep your trimmers to the lowest leaves. Do not remove anything above the bottom quarter.

It is important that you stop spraying the plants. Whatever you are using on them, be it nutrients or some other specialized chemical process, needs to stop two weeks or more before you begin the harvest. These sprays will leave a residue on the buds, and nobody wants that. Stop spraying two weeks ahead of time to prevent this from happening, and decrease the chance of mold forming on the buds. Now it's time to flush the plants.

GROWING CANNABIS

A Step-By-Step Guide to Harvesting Your Plants: Flushing

Flushing your plants is such an important part of the harvesting process that it deserves to be singled out. Flushing is done to remove any residual traces of the chemical or nutrient sprays that you used on the plants as they were growing. One of the reasons that people use marijuana these days and a key reason it is growing in popularity is the fact that it is a natural product and not chemically produced in a lab. The last thing anybody wants is to consume chemicals they didn't sign up for. It wouldn't be enjoyable for them, and it wouldn't look good for you or your product. Flushing is the easiest way to tackle this problem before it ever goes anywhere.

You might think that nobody would notice if there was residual traces of chemicals on your marijuana, but to a person experienced in consuming cannabis, it is as clear as can be. The taste of the smoke is different than it should be, harsher. Smoke with chemical traces on it burns the throat and lungs more and has a distant chemical smell. If you are growing organically, you might be able to get away without flushing, but if you are using any kind of synthetic fertilizer at all, then you absolutely must flush your plants. I recommend that you flush even if you are going straight organic because it is better to be safe than to be sorry.

Flushing your plants is going to take anywhere between a week to a week and a half. Two weeks before your planned harvest, stop spraying your plants and begin flushing them. Doing so forces the plant to use up excess nutrient it has already stored instead of taking up more from the soil. To flush, your plants simply start spraying them down, preferably with distilled water. If you have to use tap water then you can purchase a flushing agent to mix in to create your spray. If you are growing in soil (indoor or outdoor) then you spray them down with clean water just as you would spray them down with the earlier treatments. If you are running a hydroponic setup, then you just switch out the reservoir with a clean water reservoir and let it circulate for three days. After three days, empty the reservoir and fill it back up with clean water again. Do this two or three time.

If you are flushing soil then you want to have about 15% run off, give or take 5%. You should also let the plants remain dry for a day or two before you harvest as doing so will help with the drying process. If you are using a hydroponic setup then you want to take out your PPM or EC meter and check the concentration of the reservoir when flushing. If the counts are close to what they were when you had the nutrient mix then you are going to want to keep emptying and replacing the reservoir with clear water until the numbers come back down.

Doing this takes time and effort but it ensures that you do not sell or consume tainted marijuana.

A Step-By-Step Guide to Harvesting Your Plants: Harvesting

GROWING CANNABIS

It's time to actually start harvesting and bringing in the plants finally. Double check your environment. You want to avoid strong lights, temperatures above 80°F, friction from how you handle the plants, and overly damp or humid conditions. These are all harmful to the THC concentration. As the THC is the whole reason many people are looking to buy your crop, you want to make sure not to damage it this close to the finish line.

There are two ways that you can cut the plants to begin the actual harvest. The first way to to harvest the whole plant. This is the quicker of the two methods. It is also the easiest because it doesn't require that you analyze the buds beforehand. Just take the main stem and cut it off. You then take the whole plant and hang it up on your lines, or alternatively, you can cut it into smaller pieces and hang these.

The other way is to harvest the ripest buds only. This is a longer process because you need to examine all the buds in the process. Taking what you learned about the maturity of the buds, examine your plants and remove only those that are in the proper window of effect. Then, about a week later, return to the plants to harvest the buds that have matured since the last cut. The rule of thumb here is to start with the buds on the outside, those that have been exposed to the most light, as these mature faster than the ones in the shade. Doing this method takes a lot longer and requires you to examine and get to know the buds, but it can also increase the quality and size of your yield.

Put on your work gloves, they're not coming off until the rest of this is done.

Regardless of which method you use, you will find yourself looking to cut through the main stalk at one point or another. This is where your cutting tool comes in. The big fan leaves, which have no trichomes, can be removed from the plant. You might want to do this in order to make it easier for the plants to dry. If your workspace or drying space has high humidity then getting rid of the leaves is a good idea to help prevent mold from taking hold. A low humidity environment might be best if you want to leave the leaves on the drying plant.

After cutting the plants, hanging them will make it easier for them to dry in an even manner. In addition to checking the humidity, you want to make sure the area where the plants are hanging has good ventilation. Setting up fans or air conditioners can help ensure good airflow in your space.

GROWING CANNABIS

A Step-By-Step Guide to Harvesting Your Plants: Trimming

To harvest your plants, you cut them down and hung them up. Now it's time to give your plants a manicure, or trim, so you can see the buds in all their glory. Some people dry their buds on the line first, while others get to trimming right away.

If you start with trimming, then you will find that the plants dry faster once they get up on the line. Right after you cut the plants down and bring them into your harvest area, you can identify the leaves that need to be trimmed because they will be filled with water. These leaves are firm and easy to cut. You should note that the trichomes are less likely to be knocked off at this point when you are handling the buds. This is because they have become more malleable. However, a trim tray can help you to catch what does fall off, and these can be used or sold later. If you trim your plants right away, the drying process will be shorter. This quick-drying method is one to consider if you need to have the plants dried quickly for some reason or if the location is too humid. If you are a low humidity environment, however, then it is a better idea to dry first and then trim because quick-dried buds in a low humidity may become harsh when smoked.

Drying the plants is very easy, but time consuming. Hang the plants up. You will find that after three to ten days, the stems have begun to warp and break slightly. When you see this, you will know that it is time to trim the buds. Dried leaves and branches are easy to trim off at this point because they pretty much just snap right off. However, the trichomes are also more likely to fall off. You can pretty much expect to lose a lot of trichomes at this point, so again it is a good idea to have a trim tray underneath.

Regardless of whether or not you dried or trimmed first, the trimming process remains the same. Use one hand to pick up the bud and maneuver it while using the other hand to cut away any leaves and branches. You may choose to do a tight trim really close to the buds, or you may choose to leave some filler there. If you are selling the buds to be smoked or consumed, then customers are going to expect a tight trim. Marijuana is sold by weight, and customers will not want to be paying for stems, which have no effect. So remove any large leaves sticking from the buds, along with any brown or yellow leaves. If a leaf doesn't have any trichomes on it, then you can get rid of it altogether.

There are a lot of tools that can help make your trim as easy as possible. Curved trimmers are fantastic for getting in and around the circular shape of a lot of the buds. There are also bowl trimmers, which have turning cranks that allow you to toss the bud inside and turn the crank to handle the trimming.

Take your time when you first start trimming. Do not just go in waving your clippers every which way. You will end up hacking up your bud and lose money in the process. It is better to start slow and get a feel for what is and isn't worth keeping. Razors are also a useful item to have around so that you can clean off your scissors, since they'll end up getting covered in sticky residue that can slow you down or clog up your scissors.

A Step-By-Step Guide to Harvesting Your Plants: Curing

GROWING CANNABIS

Curing is a prolonged period of drying that can greatly improve your product. Plants create THCA and cannabinoids through a process called biosynthesis. Biosynthesis is a process in which some compounds are converted into new blends. For example, THCA turns into THC. You might think this process stops when you cut the plant down, but in reality, the biosynthesis process continues after harvest. By putting the freshly harvested plants into 60°F to 70°F temperatures with a humidity level of about 50%, you will provide an environment in which THCA will continue to convert into THC. Do note that if you choose to go with the quick-drying method described above, then the biosynthesis process stops earlier than if you do not.

We talked about how terpenes provide the smell and flavor in Chapter Two. These terpenes are highly volatile and will quickly degrade or even evaporate entirely at temperatures of 70°F or higher. The slow-curing method helps keep these terpenes in place so that the marijuana continues to have its aromatic elements. The conditions for curing are also ideal for enzymes and aerobic bacteria to thrive, which breaks down minerals and sugars that arise from the decomposition of chlorophyll throughout the drying process. These elements can also cause the harsh and unpleasant taste and burning that quickly-dried marijuana often has. Curing also allows the cannabinoids to stay in place (without any worry about mold!) for a couple years before any loss of potency.

So you harvested your plants, cut the branches into 12 to 16 inch pieces, removed useless leaves, and then hung them on your wire. Keep them hung up in a dark room with the previously mentioned environmental conditions alongside a fan to keep the air gently circulating. You may also want to use a dehumidifier or air conditioner to ensure that the environment stays within these ranges. This first drying will need anywhere from five to fifteen days, after which the dried buds can be cured.

To cure your buds, first trim and dry the plants as described before. Here's where things get different. Take the trimmed buds and stick them into an airtight container. It is common to see mason or canning jars used for this, but anything airtight will work. You want the buds to be loosely packed into the containers rather than filling it all up. This is done so the buds aren't crushed in the process. Pack in some of the leaves you trimmed off. Seal the containers once they are full, and store them in a dark spot. You will want it to be cool and dry. After a day, you will notice that the buds have regained some moisture and are less "crunchy." This is because the remaining moisture in the flowers have rehydrated the bud. If this doesn't happen, then your plants were overdried earlier.

After canning your buds, you are going to want to open the containers a few times each day for the next seven days. This is done to allow them to breath. Basically, moisture will leave and oxygen will rush in. If you smell ammonia when you first open a container, then you underdried the plants. The smell arises from the anaerobic bacteria eating the organic matter, and you will likely find mold or rot on your buds as well. If you find that you underdried your plants and this situation occurs, you will have to throw out the buds. If not, after that first week, you can switch to opening the jar every other day or so instead of multiple times a day. In two or three weeks, you will find that the marijuana has cured enough to have a high quality. However, if you wait four or five weeks, then you will find it to be even better off. Some strains may even be best when cured half a year or more!

This simple step is often ignored, primarily because it slows down how quickly growers can sell or consume their product, but it is how you get the absolute best buds possible from your harvest.

GROWING CANNABIS

Chapter Summary

- Harvesting lets you calculate how much your yield is worth and start the process of either enjoying or selling your product. For many growers, harvesting is the only part of the process they truly care about.

- When you harvest your crop will determine how potent and what kind of effect the bud will have.

- The amount of THC in the bud is determined by the color of the trichomes, which are little specks of white crystal on the bud that holds the THC.

- Translucent trichomes aren't mature yet and do not have enough THC to interest buyers.

- Cloudy trichomes are ready to be harvested and will provide a heady high.

- Amber trichomes are overripe but will provide a body-focused high to the user.

- If you want for cloudy trichomes to start turning amber then you can get a high that is both body and mind and can be worth a lot of money.

- Trichomes should be checked under a microscope, a pocket scope makes for a great tool in this so you do not have to take the bud off the plant.

GROWING CANNABIS

- Prepare the harvest area. You want it to be 70F degrees or less.

- Make sure you have gloves, a cutting tool, ropes to hang the plants and a trim tray.

- Cut away any old leaves left on the plants, focusing on those that are the lowest as they just steal away energy from the bud.

- Stop spraying your plants two weeks before harvesting.

- Flushing your plants means to spray them with water to clean off any chemicals that may be on them. Start flushing a week before you plan to harvest. For plants in soil you spray them as often as your treatments. For hydroponics you switch out the reservoir with clean water every three days.

- Avoid strong lights when harvesting.

- You can cut the whole plant down when you harvest or you can harvest the ripest buds first and let the others wait a week before harvesting. Cutting the whole plant is faster but with a smaller yield, the other takes much more time.

- Cut down the plants and hang them up on your lines to dry.

- Trim away the leaves and stem, cleaning up the buds. Anything without trichomes can be cut away.

- Hang the plants up to dry. Drying before trimming makes for easier trim. Trimming before drying makes for quicker dry.

- Curing your buds by drying them properly and then storing them in containers to maintain their freshness. Curing takes more time to accomplish but makes your bud much richer.

In the next chapter, you will learn about the many annoying problems you may find yourself having to tackle to keep your plants healthy and pest-free. Pests, fungi, and mold are all dangers that growers must keep in mind and be vigilant against when raising their crops.

CHAPTER EIGHT

MAINTENANCE AND PREVENTATIVE CONTROL

From planting the seeds to harvesting the plants, the journey that you have taken in this book so far has explored the best-case scenario of growing cannabis. Unfortunately, there are many steps to maintaining the health and wellbeing of your plants. Pests, fungi, and mold are all threats that can easily destroy your crop if you aren't careful.

The best approach to maintaining and defending your crops from harm is to take a preventative approach. Rather than wait for your plants to be afflicted by one of the following annoyances, take preventative steps to keep them from taking up home on your plants in the first place. This will save you the time, money and frustration that comes from battling a major infestation.

Pests

GROWING CANNABIS

There are a shocking number of pests that like to feed off of the cannabis plant. These range from large to small, some easy to spot and others masters of camouflage. Hopefully you will never have to encounter any of the following bugs.

Aphids: These are soft-bodied green, white, yellow, red, black, or brown bugs found all over the world. Baby aphids look like little white lines moving around on the leaves of your plants. They normally grow into round green or yellow creatures, but aphids infesting marijuana plants have been known to grow into black ones as well. Aphids can grow wings, and this has lead some growers into thinking they had an infestation of flies rather than aphids.

To eat, aphids stab cannabis leaves with their mouths and suck out the juices found on the inside. They like to make their homes on the underside of the leaves, so one way of spotting them is to run a paper towel or piece of toilet paper under your leaves and see if it comes away with streaks of blood. You can tell that one of your plants is dealing with a serious aphid problem when its leaves change into a yellow color and then begins to wilt.

An aphid infestation begins when winged aphids arrive, looking for a place to lay eggs. These pregnant scouts might not eat from the plant and so seem harmless, but they are usually the warning sign of a coming infestation. Preventing aphids isn't easy, especially if you grow your plants outdoors. Aphids take just a little over a week to mature, so they can quickly take up home. To get rid of them, you have to regularly look for signs of infestation and remove the bugs as soon as you see them. You can additionally use an insecticidal soap or even neem oil to get rid of them. Ladybugs eat aphids, and introducing them to your garden is a good preemptive measure to take. In addition, make sure to remove ants, as some species are known to farm aphids and deliberately increase their numbers.

Barnacle Scales: These weird-looking bugs like to take up a spot on the stems of the cannabis plant and then stop moving. They bite down into the stem and then start to weaken the plant by eating the juices inside. In doing so, the plant releases a substance called honeydew (which Aphids also love) that can attract ants and lead to mold patches on your plants. This means that the barnacle scales weaken the plant, increasing the risk of aphid infestation and mold, all at the same time.

GROWING CANNABIS

These insects do not move around a lot, so they can be a little hard to spot. To make it more challenging for the grower, barnacle scales can also blend in and look like part of the plant itself. If you spot anything on your plant that looks a little odd, give it a splash with some water and see what happens. You want to use a water sprayer to knock the scales away. Follow this up by washing the plant with insecticidal soap and neem oil like you would for aphids. You may also want to introduce ladybugs, lady beetles, or lacewings into the garden to eat the scales.

Note that the scales reproduce very quickly, so they can easily double or triple in number in no time at all. This makes them a significant threat, because they take up hold and open your plants up for all sorts of other issues. Even worse, barnacle scales do not cause any noticeable symptoms themselves. They make it easier for other creatures while hiding out and moving as little as possible. This makes them an annoying but dangerous pest.

Broad Mites: Broad mites are microscopic, and sometimes hard to spot even when they are held under a microscope. The big problem with broad mites is that because you cannot easily see them, the symptoms of their infestation are often thought to be stress, heat, overwatering, an imbalanced pH, or problems with the root. Symptoms of broad mites include new growths sticking off your plants that are twisted and droop weirdly, leaves that look wet or covered in blisters, or leaves that have the edges all turned up and wrong. Broad mites can also kill your buds when your plants begin to flower. These effects are uniform across the plant, but will always be worse in the spots where the infestation has been centralized.

The main way that people realize they have an infestation of broad mites is when they notice the damage these pests have caused. Since you cannot see them with your eyes, observing the damage is really the only way to clue into them. Their symptoms may look a lot like the effects of the tobacco mosaic virus.

Broad mites can be tricky to get rid of since many of the miticides out there aren't very good at killing them. Despite their size, broad mites are very tough. You have to cut away any part of the plant that has been infected. Any treatment you use to kill them should be used multiple times a day, and always spray the plants before you turn off the lights. You should continue any treatment you use for at least five weeks, even if you see signs of improvement in the plant before that. Broad mites can seem like they disappeared, only to show up again in a hurry because there was still one or two of them left. If you want to go the organic route and use a predator to lower the population, then you can add neoseiulus mites which prey on broad mites, into your garden.

Caterpillars and Inchworms: Caterpillars and pests like them leave some of the easiest to spot signs of their presence. If you start spotting large pieces of your leaves missing, then your first thought should be caterpillars. Clumps of brown stuff that looks like dirt on the leaves, or caterpillar poop, will confirm the infestation. Be aware that while caterpillars and inchworms look very similar, most worm-like pests on your plants are going to fall into the same categories as far as damage and treatment are concerned.

Getting rid of caterpillars is best done by using a biological insecticide such as Caterpillar BT Spray. This spray uses a bacteria called *Bacillus thuringiensis* to kill the caterpillar larva. It also makes it so that caterpillars cannot eat the cannabis leaves. The best part of using BT Spray is that though it focuses on caterpillar elimination, it also is known for killing fungus, gnats, and moths. However, BT Spray will not harm many of the beneficial insects you add to your garden. Start using BT spray as soon as you spot evidence of caterpillars on your plants, be it from damage, poop, or catching them in the act. Use it weekly.

It's always best to prevent pests from taking hold when you have the chance. If you want to avoid caterpillars then you need to start thinking of butterflies and moths as the enemy of your plants. While a butterfly on your plant might make for a beautiful picture, butterflies actually lay eggs on the plants. So while you are reaching for the camera, they may be dropping off an infestation of caterpillars that will eat your plants. Shoo those critters off whenever you see them.

Crickets: One of the loudest of the pests, you will pretty much be able to tell if you have a cricket infestation from the noise alone. You will also be able to clearly notice the damage they leave, since they chew little holes through the leaves. You can even find mole crickets attacking your plants down by the root. One or two crickets can very quickly become a major infestation as they breed very fast. However, crickets do not go after cannabis plants as much as grasshoppers or scales.

If you think that you have a cricket infestation, then you should check the plants at night, since crickets are nocturnal creatures. They are attracted to lights at night, and so turning them off to match the sun's natural schedule can help you avoid them. They are also attracted to the messiness of unclean leaf litter and biological waste; even the garbage can draw them in. You can use cricket traps to capture them, but if you have a full blown infestation, these traps will only help to reduce their numbers, not solve the problem as a whole. Insecticidal soap and neem oil are again very useful. You may also consider using a floating row cover to prevent crickets from having access to the plants. This netting goes over your plants, but still allows water and sunlight to get through to the plant. Floating row covers are useful in preventing pests, but can be an annoyance to use.

Fungus Gnats: Gnats have the appearance of small flies. They enjoy spending time in the soil around your plants, as their young like to grow in wet soil before moving up to the surface to snack on your plants. Gnats show up often on plants that are overwatered, so the first step you should take in prevention is to ensure that you are watering your plants in a healthy manner. When watering your plants, let the top inch of the soil dry out before you water them again. Doing so will leave the gnats without the moist soil they need to raise their young, in which case they will move on to other plants. This practice also helps in getting rid of an infestation but it can take weeks to work.

GROWING CANNABIS

First check for fungus gnats by using your eyes to spot the bugs themselves. The gnats will be visible before any damage is, so they are their own warning sign. As soon as you spot the gnats, examine your watering habits and see if you should be slowing down. Adult gnats do not do much damage to your plants as larvae do, but they can still spread diseases, which could then absolutely devastate a crop. However, the real danger is in the larvae they leave in your soil. Though these creatures are tiny, they feed primarily on the roots of the cannabis plant, which will weaken the plants and can cause serious damage if not contained.

If you are having problems with fungus gnat larvae, then you will notice what is called a "damping off" of the seeds. Seedlings may appear to just be weak, without any real sign as to why they are just dropping dead. Adult plants slowly start to wilt and turn yellow with nasty spots all over them. The leaves will appear as if they have a nutrient deficiency or as if the pH level was causing a problem. The growth of your plants will slow down and maybe even stop, and the yield of your plants will be lower than normal.

Taking care of the watering issue is the first step in dealing with gnats and their sticky larvae, but you may want to use sticky traps down by your roots. Yellow-colored traps, in particular, are highly effective as gnats are drawn to the color. The glue on the trap will keep gnats stuck and help kill off the population. It also is a great way of seeing just how bad the infestation is, since the more gnats in the trap, the bigger the problem. A fan blowing over your plants and soil can be beneficial as well, since it keeps the soil dry and makes it more difficult to fly around. Larvae in the soil can be killed with neem oil, and sprinkling diatomaceous earth over the top of the soil is a great approach to prevent further issues.

Grasshoppers and Locusts: These annoying critters love the taste of cannabis leaves. They will chew right through the leaves and then start living on the branches of your plant with an attitude like they just started paying you rent. They'll eat the stems as well, which can kill entire branches of your plants. This makes them an absolutely deadly pest, more than capable of killing off a crop if left unchecked. They need to be dealt with quickly, or else they can leave you miserable.

Check for grasshopper infestations often. In fact, you should really be checking your plants for signs of any infestation on a daily basis, just to stay safe and vigilant. Spinosad products, which kill grasshoppers on touch, can be sprayed over the plants to reduce their numbers. Spinosad products are harmless to humans, pets, and plants, as they are made from the fermented actinomycete *Saccharopolyspora spinosa*. *S. spinosa* is a soil bacterium that causes the grasshoppers to die after ingestion by destroying their nervous systems. Insecticidal soaps and neem oil are effective here as well, as with many of the various pests you will encounter. Floating row covers help prevent grasshoppers, too, as the insects are too big to squeeze under the covers.

Leafhoppers: These little guys chew on the leaves of the cannabis plant, and in turn, leave the leaves covered in brown and yellow spots that resemble acne. Leafhoppers are also known for spreading disease, and this makes them particularly dangerous to your crops. There are many, many different kinds of leafhoppers. In fact, there are more than 20,000 identifiable types. This means that leafhoppers come in all shapes and sizes, though the most common type is the *Graphocephala coccinea*. Otherwise known as the candy striped leafhopper, these little colorful bugs would be beautiful to look at if they were not so dangerous. Leafhoppers like to eat your plants when the atmosphere is dry, since they are after the moisture in the cannabis leaves.

The spots that leafhoppers leave behind will be concentrated into small clusters. These insects suck sap from the leaves, which changes the leaf color in that location. They do not chew holes through leaves themselves, but rather just leave them looking gross and damaged. With so many different types of leafhoppers, they can look very different from one another. But all leafhoppers share a few attributes. Leafhoppers are insects, so they have six legs; they also all have wings and move by jumping and sliding. They also all die the same way, which is a great benefit to us growers.

Check your plants for signs of leafhoppers. If the atmosphere is dry then you should be checking for the little pests more often, as this is when they are the thirstiest. They like to hide on the underside of leaves, since they do not like to be caught snacking. Use spinosad products and follow with insecticidal soap and neem oil. Leafhoppers are food to lady beetles (such as ladybugs), lacewings, and parasitic wasps. These bugs will each eat quite a lot of leafhoppers, so releasing them can be a great way to reduce their numbers. They are also slowed down by floating row covers but these only work for prevention, not reduction of an already established infestation.

Leaf Miners: By far one of the weirdest pests that you can find yourself dealing with, the leaf miner actually lives inside of the cannabis leaf, rather than eating it or chewing on the outside like most other pests. Leaf miners open up the leaf to enter inside, and then they start to mine their way through it. This lets them eat the most delicious pieces of the leaves. You will be able to spot them inside your leaves as they bulge out. They also leave a trail of damage behind them that could look like zigzagging white lines that run through the leaves. Leaf miners aren't so much a single species of pests as they are a catchall term for many different pests that use the leaves as a home and snack bar.

GROWING CANNABIS

The first step in getting rid of a leaf miner problem is to cut away any of the leaves that have already been affected. If you have started to see the tell tale lines of damage they leave behind, then you should cut away these leaves immediately. This is highly unlikely to fix the problem outright, but it can reduce the number of leaf miners in the plant. You can crush the larva inside of the leaf itself if you are nervous about cutting them off. Spinosad is useful here, as is neem oil. A BT spray may help if the leaf miners are caterpillar larvae. Another option, after getting some floating row covers to reduce infection, is to release some *Diglyphus isaea* into your garden. These are parasitic wasps that will kill and eat leaf miners for you. These wasps like other pests too, and will eat them as well, but they'll eventually fly away after a few days, in which case you will have to purchase and release more.

Mealybugs: These bugs are covered in white hair that makes them look kind of like mold. Many growers see them and think they have a mold problem, and so they then treat their plants for the wrong issue. Mealybugs love warm temperatures and absolutely hate the cold. Worse, they do not just go after your plants while they're growing. Mealybugs can be found on your plants after harvest, making them one of the pests that hold on the longest. The patches they leave can look like mold, powder, or even the webbing of a spider. Just like scales and aphids, these bugs suck out honeydew from the cannabis plants, an act that leaves your plant susceptible to soot, mold, or ants (which makes the aphid problems worse). Mealybugs look like white versions of scales, except that they move a lot.

An infestation of mealybugs is going to be a pain to get rid of. Insecticidal soaps help in this regard, but as mealybugs are highly resilient critters, it is best to try more than one brand or method of elimination when tackling them. It will likely take constant treatment to get rid of mealybugs, but, as tempting as it might be, you should not use all of your chemicals at one. Rotate them one at a time instead. If you are using insecticidal soap on Monday, then you would use neem oil on Tuesday, for example. First, however, you should start by using a water spray to remove as many of the mealybugs as you can see. This is a step you can take every day, but combine it with a process like neem oil rather than use the water spray to replace a day's step. When it comes to insecticidal soaps, it is best to find one that has a high concentration of fatty acid salts because these weaken the outer shell of the mealybug without damaging the plants or leaving behind a trace. Neem oil helps, but never get the stuff on your buds. Alcohol is actually a great way to kill them and you can either use a cotton swab to kill the bugs individually or you can mix rubbing alcohol with water to make a spray. Just keep it at nine to one water to alcohol mixture.

Of course, mealybugs are also super tasty to lady beetles, ladybugs, and lacewings, so these insects can be highly useful if you find you have a mealybug problem. Diatomaceous earth will work as well. This stuff is made from fossilized shells so it is very, very sharp when you look at it on the microscopic scale. This allows it to stab into and through the exoskeleton of pests, making them bleed out and lose the fluids inside of them, but it is too small to do any damage to larger animals like pets or children. In fact, while it would be gross, it could even be eaten without causing harm. Not that it is recommended, of course.

Slugs and Snails: These little guys love eating the leaves of your cannabis plants and even chewing on the buds. You may notice trails of slime on your plants that leads to or away from damage and holes that have scalloped edges. The bite marks from slugs and snails looks quite similar to the damage left by caterpillars. You will know it is slugs and snails instead of caterpillars if the edges of the damaged parts begin to look smooth. Like crickets, these pests are most active at night. They are more likely to appear in spring, and can come out earlier than many of the other pests. If they are attacking seedlings, then you shouldn't be surprised to see entire seedlings die overnight thanks to these little guys.

To deal with slugs and snails, you could allow frogs or beetles, their natural predators, into the garden. But even better than killing slugs and snails off after they've set up shop is to prevent the infestation by making it impossible for the slugs to reach your plants. You can do so by taking a plastic bottle, cutting it in half widthwise, and then using each half as a wall or makeshift greenhouse to cover a seedling. Another approach is to sprinkle lime, eggshells, diatomaceous earth, or sawdust in a circle around the plant. The slugs and snails will not be able to cross that barrier to get at your plant without killing themselves. Slugs seem to love plates, orange rings, and beer. Fill a pot with some beer, and you can find slugs that dropped in and drowned themselves in the brew.

A really effective beer trap can be made by taking some flour and some stale beer and mixing them together in a container. Set this in your garden with the top a couple centimeters from the ground so that the slugs and snails can easily climb into the container. If you do not have beer, then you can use wine, juice, yeasty water, or even sugar water as the liquid part of the trap instead. The flour thickens the liquid and makes it almost impossible for the pests to escape. You can expect these traps to fill up often, so remember to check them on a daily basis.

Spider Mites: As suggested by their name, spider mites are part of the same overarching family that gives us spiders and ticks. They're one of the more common pests when it comes to cannabis crops. Unfortunately, they're also one that latches on hard and is hard to drive off. These pests have really sharp mouths which they use to bite into the cannabis plant and suck out its liquid. The leaves of your plants are left covered in tiny, bump-like yellow, orange, or white specks. Spider mites are more common when you are using a soil-based growing method, though they can still infect a hydroponic setup. One of the biggest problems with these pests is their small size, which allows them to really populate a crop before a grower notices them.

These pests reproduce quickly, seem to disappear only to come back a few days later, eat large volumes of plant matter, cover your plants in gross silk webbing that can further damage crops, and survive almost anything you throw at them. That's the worst part with them—spider mites quickly grow immune to your chemical solutions, so you need to switch up what you use to drive them off. Otherwise, they learn to ignore it. If you are growing indoors, then spider mites were most likely transmitted to your plants because you forgot to clean yourself off before you started working on your crop.

If you have an infestation of spider mites, then you will want to lower the heat and get some fans blowing on your plants. Spider mites like warmth, and they hate the wind, so make them regret making your plants their new home. You can spray water on them to knock them off as well. Next, use Azamax in small amounts with your watering to kill any mites that are in the soil. Spinosad should be used, along with Essentria IC3 insecticide, which is often used to kill bed bugs. Insecticidal soaps with fatty acid salts will help. You will even want to get a specialized product like Dokto Doom Spider Mite Knockout Spray. Seriously, eradicating spider mites takes a lot of work because of their high immunity. Ladybugs and predatory mites may also help, along with diatomaceous earth. Remember to treat the entire growing area, all of your soil, and everything. They do not just hang out on the plants.

Only use one of the above chemical solutions at a time. Use one solution, wait two days, and then use another one. Keep this up until you think all of the spider mites are gone. Then do it again, repeating so that you use each of your chemical solutions once more. Spider mites are notorious for sticking around long after you thought they left, so it is better to play it safe than to be sorry.

GROWING CANNABIS

Thrips: It really is annoying how so many of these pests are really tiny. Thrips are no different here. They are small and quick when adults but tiny and still when young. There are many different types of thrips. Some are gold with wings, others are dark, and some are wormy. No matter how they look, thrips all want to chew your leaves and suck out their insides to leave silver and bronze patches all over. The damage they leave looks similar to the damage made by spider mites, except a lot bigger and less uniform in shape. If left unchecked, then thrips will soon kill off the leaves they're eating.

You're going to want to start treating the plants with insecticidal soap and make sure that you avoid any buds on the plant. Next comes the neem oil so that the pests find that your plants taste horrible, making them want to move on to tastier treats. Spinosad should come after that, so you can kill off a bunch of the thrips on contact. Another insecticide you can use for thrips is pyrethrins. However, pyrethrins are toxic to bees and some mammals, and so should only be used if you have no other options remaining. Hopefully, you will not need to worry about pyrethrins, as thrips are not nearly as hard to get rid of as spider mites are.

Whiteflies: The last of the pests, these ones look like white moths but act very similarly to spider mites. As with many other pests, they tend to collect on the bottom of leaves to suck their meal out. But though whiteflies eat on the bottom, it is the top of the leaf that starts to show white spots. You will likely notice the pests themselves, as their white color stands out against the green of the cannabis plant. Because of the way they flutter and move, you will most likely notice them before you notice the damage. Shake the plant and see if any whiteflies start to flutter around. This is the clearest sign in the world that you have an infestation on your hands. They lay eggs onto the leaves with a sticky residue that makes it almost impossible to wipe them off. This lets a population get out of hand quickly.

Start with your insecticidal soap and then move onto the neem oil. From there you can move into spinosad. Essentria IC3 is useful in killing off whiteflies when used daily. You need to treat your plants often as whiteflies can flutter away from the plant during treatment and land on another part that hasn't yet been attacked. The shifting nature of an infestation of whiteflies can make for a very annoying battle, so always be careful to treat all of your plants and not just the parts with the heaviest concentrations.

Fungi and Molds

Fungi show up when the humidity around your plants is too high or when your plants have been weakened by pests. Unlike pests, fungi do not move around and make themselves noticed. They instead show up suddenly and silently. Fungi might take some time getting settled but can spread quickly.

Prevention is better than treatment, so ensure that you are always following proper hygiene rules when dealing with your plants. Always disinfect the area between crops and clean your hands and clothes before entering the grow room. Always remove dead plant matter from around your crops as these grow, since the decomposition attracts fungi. You want to make sure the temperature stays in healthy ranges for the plants rather than the fungi. You can purchase organic products with fungicidal properties.

One common type of fungus is botrytis, or gray mold. This pathogenic fungus is easy to detect, but spreads quickly and can kill a plant in a couple of days. Look for the brown and gray, dry texture. Cut off any infected part, taking a little bit of the healthy plant nearby to be safe.

Powdery mildew is a white, dust-like fungus that covers the leaves and buds of your plants. It's not very lethal, but should still be removed, so discard any infected areas and use fungicide on your plants.

Mildew will take hold on leaves, stems, or flowers. It is found on the underside of the plant and can be spotted because of the yellow stains it leaves on your leaves. If you notice yellow stains and white dust, then you have mildew. The first thing to do is to create better ventilation for the plants by cutting away the infected areas and opening up the plant to breathe better. Then, use your fungicide.

Fusarium is a fungus that is found not on the leaves but down in the soil. Fusarium feed on the plant until it dies by preventing sap flow inside the plant itself. When sap doesn't flow properly, the plant will start to rot at the stem, and you will notice the oldest of the leaves start to strain. This is bad news because there is no treatment for fusarium, so all there is to do is toss out the infected plants.

Chapter Summary

- Aphids are small bugs that like to hang out on the bottom of leaves and can be a pain to get rid of.

- Barnacle scales are pests that take up a spot on your plants and then do not move. While they do not do an overly lot of damage themselves, they open your plants up to wider threats.

- Broad mites are impossible to see with the naked eye and easy to misdiagnose. They're tough to kill so keep an eye out for their damage early.

- Caterpillars can absolute wreck havoc on cannabis. It is best to use a biological insecticide like Caterpillar BT spray to kill them.

- Crickets can be heard, making them easy to spot. They are attracted to messiness so keep your grow area clean.

- Fungus gnats love plants that are being overwatered. Make sure you water properly and you will probably never have to deal with them.

- Grasshoppers absolutely love eating cannabis and can kill off plants quickly.

- Leafhoppers come in all sorts of forms but they die the same. If the atmosphere is dry then you should be keeping an eye out for them.

GROWING CANNABIS

- Leaf miners live in the leaves, requiring you to cut them out and throw them away.

- Mealybugs look like mold but are one of the hardest pests to get rid of.

- Slugs or snails can be beaten with beer traps.

- Spider mites are the worst pests because they quickly grow immune to insecticides.

- Thrips can also get out of control quickly but are much easier to deal with than spider mites.

- Whiteflies can be spotted because they fly away when disturbed. Make sure to treat all of the plants and not just the most infected parts, otherwise they'll just fly to new leaves.

- Fungi and molds are silent killers that you must watch out for and treat immediately.

In the next chapter, you will learn about the most common mistakes that new growers make when they first start cultivating cannabis. Avoiding these mistakes will save you lots of time and trouble with your first crops.

CHAPTER NINE

COMMON MISTAKES TO AVOID

We looked at some of the mistakes that new growers make when it comes to cloning plants. Now it's time to look at those mistakes that are common across almost all new growers. If you can avoid falling into these harmful behaviors, then you can start your first crop with a leg up to ensure you get the best marijuana possible.

Not Bothering to Look after the pH Level

Every plant will have an optimal pH in which it best grows, but many people do not even bother trying to understand what a pH level is when they first start out. There is a ton of vocabulary that you learn when you begin growing anything, a lot of which isn't overly important. However, it is crucial that you listen to and pay attention to your growing medium's pH.

What pH does it determine just how many and which kinds of nutrients your plants will be able to use.

If you have a pH in the wrong ranges, then your plants will not be able to fully make use of the nutrients that you feed it. There is much literature about pH levels and its importance out there, but when it comes to growing marijuana, what you need to know is that cannabis grows best in a hydroponic medium when the pH is between 5.5 and 6.5 and best in a soil medium when the pH is between 6.0 and 7.0. Check your pH levels often to make sure everything is working properly.

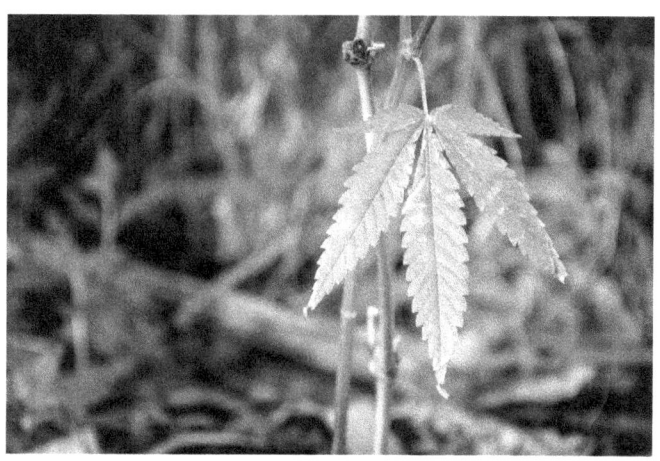

Stop Overfeeding Nutrients

Nutrients are good for us and for our plants, so more nutrients would be more good, right? While the logic seems to check out, reality tells a different picture. When you overfeed your plants with too many nutrients, they will eventually suffer from nutrient burn. It might not kill your plants, but it will leave them feeling rough and unhealthy, making them more at risk from pests.

Create a feeding schedule for your plants so that they always get their nutrients when expected. Only use a quarter or half of the recommended dosage, as many companies recommend using way more than needed. If the plant looks like it doesn't have enough nutrients but the pH is in the ranges above, then you will want to feed a little more nutrients on your next dosage.

Stop Overwatering Your Plants

Overwatering your plants is going to make them more susceptible to pests, start drooping down, and, if you are really over doing it, even die outright. Check your growing medium before watering your plants. Stick a finger in an inch and see if it is dry. If it is, then water your plants. But if it isn't, then do not water them yet. You shouldn't water them too often, only when they pass the dry check.

Control the Climate Properly

When it comes to growing cannabis, it is all about the temperature and humidity. They both need to be in the right ranges if you want your plants to really flourish. A poorly managed climate will hurt your plants more than any pest will.

Temperature needs to be just right. When it is low, your plants do not grow as quickly or as big. If the temperature is low enough then your plants will not

GROWING CANNABIS

grow at all, they'll just die instead. But if the temperature is too high, then the plants will suffer from heat stress, and you will see the leaves curl up because they are trying to get shade from the sun. If left to suffer heat stress for too long, then the plants will die. Keep the plants around 75°F.

In general, the humidity should be low. You may want a higher humidity on certain plants under specific circumstances, as with the clones we saw earlier, but for the most part, humidity is best kept low. An overly humid environment leaves your plants at risk for mold, fungi, and pests. Keep in mind that the ideal humidity should also change with the plant's life stage. A seedling might like humidity around 60% but as it grows that should be dropped down closer to 40%.

GROWING CANNABIS

Chapter Summary

- The pH level controls how many nutrients your plants can make use of.

- Cannabis should have a pH between 5.5 and 6.5 in a hydroponic system. Plants grown in soil need a pH between 6.0 and 7.0.

- Too many nutrients will cause your plants to suffer nutrient burn and this will greatly weaken them, making threats from pests even more dangerous.

- Too much water can kill plants and open them up to infection and infestation.

- Cannabis needs to be kept around 75°F degrees.

- Humidity should be around the 40% range for full-grown plants and 60% for seedlings.

FINAL WORDS

As cannabis is increasingly legalized around the world, the industry will only continue to grow. Now is the time to get onboard, to make preparations for this shift, and get in on the ground floor. With the book in your hands, you have a resource that you can return to anytime to remember how to keep your marijuana crops healthy and get the most out of them.

Cultivating cannabis is one of those fields where you can really dive in and do as little or as much as you like. The bigger your operation, the more you will make back upon harvest. But many growers only want a plant or two of their own and that's perfectly fine too. Whatever your goals are with your crops, remember to take care of them and check in with them everyday. They might just be plants but you should consider them your babies, put in the work to keep them healthy, and see them grow up into beautiful buds.

Experiment with breeding and cloning your plants to get the most potent buds you can. Maybe you will invent the next strain to win awards. You never know if you do not try.

www.ingramcontent.com/pod-product-compliance
Lightning Source LLC
Chambersburg PA
CBHW050325120526
44592CB00014B/2050